Reaching the Goal: Expanding Access to HIV Treatment for Improved Health

Khansa

First Printing, 2024

CONTENTS

ÍËHÌ ÏHĀ F GSĀÆĄĈĀČĀÇĀČÈĀ

ÍËHÌËÌĀQZČĈĀÅÁĀÀĄĆĀABÎĀ[illegible]

ÍËHÌ Ï Ā IĀÅĀVÁZĀČĄĀ OQĀČĆZV[illegible]

ÍËHÍĀ ĈĈZĈĈÅZÅČĀĄÀĀĆĀĈĀĀĄÀĀW[illegible]ĈĀË

ÍËHÎĀ ĈĈZĈĈÅZÅČĀĄÀĀĄÇ[illegible]ÈĀĄÀĀČĀZĀZÇ[illegible]

ÍËHÎĀLÇZĆ[illegible]ĀĄÀĀZÇĀ[illegible]

ÍËHÏĀBĀĈXĊĈĈĀĄÅĀ

ÍËHÏ ÏHĀ PĊÅÅVĆÈĀĄÀĀÅVĀÅĀĆZĈĊĀČĈĀ

ÍËHĪĀ PĊÅÅVĆÈĀĄÀĀZÇĀYZÅX[illegible]ĀÇZĆĈĊĈĀĈČVÅYVĆ[illegible]ĈĀÅÅĀ[illegible]

ÍËHĪ ÏHĀ RÆČVĀZĀĄ[illegible]

ÍËHĪ Ï Ā ĀFGSĀÆĄĈĀČĀÇĀČÈĀ

ÍËHĪËĀÍĀIĀÅĀVÁZĀ[illegible]

ÍËHĪ Ï Ā PĄXĀVĀÅĀVĆÅĈĀ

ÍËHĪĀPĊÅÅVĆÈĀĄÀĀZÇĀYZÅXZĒĀ[illegible]ĀĄÀĀYĀÀĀZĆZÅČĀVÆ[illegible]

ÍËHĬ ÏHĀ F GSĀÆĄĈĀČĀÇĀČÈĀ

ÍËHĬ Ï Ā QZĈČZYĀĀĄ[illegible]XĄĊÅČĀ

ÍËHĬ Ï Ā PČVĆČZYĀ [illegible]

ÍËHİĀLÇZĆV[illegible]ZÅZĈĈĀĄÀĀČĀZĀZÇĀYZÅXZĀ[illegible]

ÍËÌĤĀ NĊV[illegible]ČÈĀĄÀĀČĀZĀZÇ[illegible]

ÍËÌHĀMĄČZÅ[illegible]WĀVĈZĈĀÅÅĀČĀZĀĆZÇĀZ[illegible]

ÍËÌÌĀ ÁĆZZÅZÅĈČĀVÅYĀYĀĈVÁĆZZÅZÅĈČĀĎĀČĀÅĄČĀZĆĀĈČĊYĀ[illegible]

ÍËÌÍ Ā GÅÆĀĀXVČĀĄÅĀÀĄĆĀ[illegible]

AF MQ COĀDLRO[illegible]

ÎËĤ NĊVĀĀČVČĀÇZĀZÇĀYZÅXZĀĈ[illegible]

ÎËĤ ĀĈĖ[illegible]ÅVČ[illegible]ZÇĀ[illegible]ZĀÇ[illegible]YZÅXZĀĄ[illegible]ČĀ[illegible]ÅVW[illegible]ÅYĀYZĆĆÅĀĀ
ĊÆČVĀZĀĄ[illegible]ZĈĈĀÅĀĀĀĀ ÀĆĀXVĖ

ÎËÌĀ GÅČĆĄYĊXČ[illegible]

ÎËÍĀLWĀZXČĀ[illegible]

ÎËÎĀJ ZČĀĄYĈĀ

ÎËÎËĤ PZVĆXÂĀĈĈĈV[illegible]

ÎËĨĀGÅXĀĊĈĀĄÅĀVÅYĀZĐXĀĊĈĀĄ[illegible]

ÎËÏËĤ BVČVĀZĐĈĆVXČĀĄÅĀVÅYĀÅVÅ[illegible]

ÎËĪĀ NĊVĀĀČÈĀVĈĈZĈĈÅZÅČĀ[illegible]VĀĀČVČĀÇZĀ[illegible]

ÎËĬĀ ĈĈZĈĈÅZÅČĀĄÀĀXĄÅĀĀYZÅXZĀĀÅĀČĀZĀĆZÇ[illegible]

ÎËİĀ ÅVĀĖĈĀĈĀVÅYĀĈÈÅČĀZĈĀĈĀ[illegible]

ÎËHĤ OZĈĈ[illegible]ĈĀ

ÎËHĤËH BVČVWVĈZĀPZV[illegible]

CHAPTER ONE

1.0 General introduction and literature review

1.1 Introduction

In 2006, the UN General Assembly endorsed the continued scale-up of Human Immunodeficiency Virus (HIV) prevention, treatment, care and support aiming at universal access by 2010 (WHO/UNAIDS 2007). Maximum benefits in terms of reduced morbidity and mortality are associated with care and support. Benefits such as availability of antiretroviral therapy (ART) or cotrimoxazole and ART prophylaxis for prevention of mother–to–child transmission (PMTCT) interventions are obtained with early diagnosis (UNAIDS 2014, UNAIDS 2018).

Early diagnosis provides an opportunity to empower people living with HIV (PLHV) with information and skills to prevent HIV transmission (UNAIDS 2014, UNAIDS 2018). Furthermore, there is evidence that ART reduces the transmission of HIV through suppression of viral load among discordant couples. There is a positive correlation between increased access to ART and population-level HIV incidence; for each 10% increase in ART coverage, the population–level transmission rate decreases by 1%. Indeed, the HIV incidence is less than half in low and middle–income countries (LMICs) with high ART coverage than those with low ART coverage (UNAIDS 2014, UNAIDS 2018).

Further, existing evidence supports the fact that PLHV benefit more when ART is initiated in the early stages of HIV infection (WHO 2013). In 2010, the ART eligibility criteria were revised from CD4 cell counts of 200 to 350 cells/μl. (UNAIDS 2015). The changes increased the number of PLHV enrolled in ART by 1.5 times by the end of 2010 compared to 2008, indicating an increase in expectation and demand for ART(UNAIDS 2015). In 2011, all United Nation countries signed an agreement to combat the HIV epidemic.

The aim was to reduce by half, sexual and vertical HIV transmission, tuberculosis deaths among people with HIV and to deliver ART to 15 million people (United Nations General Assembly 2011). In 2013, the World Health Organization (WHO) recommended that the cut–off point for initiation of ART for PLHV should be a CD4 cell count of 500 based on the benefits associated with much earlier initiation of ART (WHO 2013). The current guidelines now recommend initiation of ART in all people with HIV regardless of WHO disease stage and at any CD4 cell count (UNAIDS 2015, UNAIDS 2018).

According to a 2015 UNAIDS report, the world achieved the AIDS targets of Millennium Development Goal (MDG) 6 by providing ART to 15 million people living with HIV. According to UNAIDS Executive Director Michel Sidibé: "This is the first time in the history of global health that we have reached a treatment target by the deadline". Based on this, a new target for ART has been set by UNAIDS/WHO known as '95–95–95'. By 2030: (a) 95% of all PLHIV will know their status;(b) 95% of all people with an HIV diagnosis will receive sustained ART; and (c) 95% of all people receiving ART will achieve viral suppression (UNAIDS 2015, UNAIDS 2017, UNAIDS 2018). The rationale for these targets is to end HIV/AIDS by 2030 (UNAIDS 2015, UNAIDS 2017, UNAIDS 2018).

To attain these targets, people at risk of HIV need to learn their status and be linked to HIV prevention, care and treatment. Indeed, linkage to HIV care is conditional upon knowing one's status through HIV testing. If linkage to care is not accomplished, a major goal of the provision of HIV Testing Services (HTS) fails (Wanyenze et al., 2011).

This book reports on research to develop and evaluate a behaviour change intervention (BCI) to increase HIVST uptake and linkage to HIV prevention, care and treatment among hard to reach populations in an African setting.

1.2 HIV testing and Counselling Services

HIV Testing and Counselling Services (HTS) reduce HIV transmission risk behaviours especially among individuals diagnosed with HIV and within sero discordant couples (Wanyenze et al., 2011) and is also a gateway to HIV prevention, care and treatment (Wanyenze et al., 2011). HTS is defined as a process whereby an individual or couples undergo counselling enabling them to make an informed choice on being tested for HIV (WHO/UNAIDS 2007). According to the WHO, HTS, regardless of the model of delivery, must adhere to the five Cs – Consent, Confidentiality, Counselling, Correct test results and linkage to Care (UNAIDS/WHO 2004). Mandatory or coerced testing is inappropriate, irrespective of its source whether from a health care worker or a partner or relative (UNAIDS/WHO 2004).

There are four main HTS models of delivery, of which two, Client-Initiated Testing and Counselling (CITC) and Provider-Initiated Testing and Counselling (PITC) are well accepted, feasible, effective and cost-effective at increasing coverage (Hutchinson et al., 2006, Menzies et al., 2009, WHO 2009, Waters et al., 2011).

The other two approaches are diagnostic HIV testing and mandatory HIV–testing screening (WHO 2009). It is important to mention that CITC, also known as a community–based HTS and PITC, also known as facility-based HTS, attain different testing outcomes with the community–based HTS more likely to reach and link key and vulnerable populations (KVPs) to HIV care (Suthar et al., 2013).

The evidence that the community–based HTC approach can reach KVPs underscores the importance of scaling up community-based HIV–testing services to this subgroup. According to the WHO, KVPs, also known as most–at–risk, refer to men who have unprotected sex with men (MSM) (Carballo-Dieguez et al., 2012), transgender people, people who inject drugs (PWIDs) and/or people who use drugs (PWUDs), women who engage in transactional sex, commercial sex workers (CSWs) and their clients (WHO 2008, WHO 2013).

KVPs also include miners, soldiers and long-distance lorry drivers (WHO 2013). Global statistics, however, suggest that nearly 49% of adults are unaware of their HIV status – these are mostly men, adolescent pregnant women and KVPs. In addition, there is an "a spill-over" of HIV infections from KVP into the general population, with sexual partners of KVP acting as bridging populations (UNAIDS 2015, UNAIDS 2017, UNAIDS 2018). Moreover, there are subgroups, often related to specific contexts, such as female bar workers (FBWs) and male mountain climbing porters (MCPs) in the Kilimanjaro area, who are not classified as KVPs by WHO despite exhibiting a high risk of HIV infection (Ostermann et al., 2014). Reaching such subgroups with novel HTC initiatives such as HIV Self- Testing (HIVST) is imperative for early identification and linkage to HIV prevention, care and treatment (UNAIDS 2017, UNAIDS 2018).

Early linkages to HIV prevention, care and treatment are associated with improved patient outcomes. However, there is no standard definition for linkage to HIV care for either HIV surveillance or monitoring and evaluation of HTC programmes. The concept of linkage to HIV prevention, care and treatment imply receipt of care or treatment at relevant time points (UNAIDS 2017, UNAIDS 2018). Various studies, however, define linkage differently (Gardner et al., 2005, Wanyenze et al., 2011, Govindasamy et al., 2013, Suthar et al., 2013, Naik et al., 2015). Suthar, et al. define linkage to care as (a) from HIV diagnosis to CD4 measurement and (b) from being eligible to ART to initiating ART (Suthar et al., 2013). Wanyenze, et al. define linkage to care as self–report of attendance at HIV/AIDS clinic post-diagnosis.

Gardner, et al. define linkage to care as self–report of attendance at HIV care provider at least once in two consecutive six–month time periods (Metsch et al., 2005). Govindasamy, et al. define linkage to care as newly diagnosed HIV–infected subjects who visit the clinic to see health providers at the health facility at least once after diagnosis within specific durations post-diagnosis. The durations are defined as within 1, 3 and 6 months for patients with CD4 counts$\leq$ 200, 350 or greater than or equal to 350 cell/μl respectively (Kranzer et al., 2013). Naik, et al. define linkage to care as obtaining CD4 count post-diagnosis (Doherty et al., 2015).

1.3 Characteristics of different HIV testing services

Globally, diverse models of HIV testing services (HTS) are in use and innovations in HIV–testing approaches are continually being developed to increase uptake of HIV testing and linkage to HIV prevention, care and treatment. A WHO guideline on the use of antiretroviral drugs for treating and preventing HIV infection summarises diverse models of HTS and underscores the importance of HIV testing as an opportunity for more people to access HTS and know their HIV status (WHO 2013, UNAIDS 2017, UNAIDS 2018). CITC, which is often termed as voluntary counselling and testing (VCT), was the earliest HTS delivery model to promote increased access to testing. Primarily offered in freestanding VCT centres, but also within clinical settings, CITC had been a prominent approach. Evidence from studies on CITC in different settings has shown an increase in uptake of HTS, coverage of HTS and identification of first–time testers (Sweat 2000, Sweat et al., 2011, Sweat et al., 2012).

Another approach recommended by WHO in health facilities is PITC, whereby health care providers offer HIV testing and counselling to all clients, including pregnant women attending health facilities to reach more HIV–positive people, who may need more medical attention. Evidence from studies on PITC testing in different settings has shown an increase in the identification of new HIV positive patients among the previous non–testers (Obermeyer and Osborn 2007, Suthar et al., 2013).

Diagnostic HIV testing is a screening procedure to aid clinical diagnosis and clinical management of patients with HIV–related signs and symptoms, including all tuberculosis patients. Finally, a mandatory HIV–testing screening approach is offered in clinical settings for HIV and other blood-borne viruses, such as Hepatitis, for all blood and organ transplant donors (WHO 2009, UNAIDS 2017, UNAIDS 2018).

Expanding access to HTS is imperative to increase rates of HIV testing and early identification of PLHIV. Early identification of newly diagnosed HIV–positive individuals will facilitate linkage to care and initiation of ART and reduce HIV transmission (UNAIDS 2017, UNAIDS 2018).

A home-based Voluntary Testing and Counselling (HBVCT) provide HTS delivery within the home environment. Two primary models for conducting HBVCT service delivery are (a) testing offered 'door–to–door' and provided to consenting individuals; and (b) index testing via a known or suspected HIV or TB–positive index patient to others within their households. Another version of HBVCT is couple home-based Voluntary Testing and counselling (cHBVCT) (Allen et al., 2003, Bateganya et al., 2008, Njau et al., 2012, UNAIDS 2017, UNAIDS 2018).

Mobile or outreach testing models provide service delivery within community settings through mobile vans or tents or organized testing events. The testing model might deliver services through community sites such as churches or schools, or events, including sporting events, by stand-alone VCT service providers. Evidence has shown that mobile or outreach HTS increase access to HTS for hard–to–reach populations, particularly in rural settings, previously undiagnosed men, mobile populations, such as miners and populations with a higher risk of HIV exposure (Morin et al., 2006, Kranzer et al., 2012, UNAIDS 2017, UNAIDS 2018).

Workplace and school-based VCT delivery models provide HTS within a workplace or school. The strategy aims to provide services to individuals who have limited access to other services due to formal employment (often men), or who have high opportunity costs associated with seeking HTS due to educational commitments (Corbett et al., 2006). Lastly, the HIVST model provides individuals with an opportunity to test for HIV in the environment of their choice.

There is increasing evidence that HIVST has the potential to empower at high–risk individuals, such as health care workers to test for HIV (Choko et al., 2011, MacPherson et al., 2011, Kebede et al., 2013, Kalibala et al., 2014, Kumwenda et al., 2014, WHO 2016). Table 1.1 presents a summary of the different HTS models.

able 1.1. Four types of HTS delivery models recommended by WHO

Approach	Description	Service-delivery model
Client–initiated Testing &Counselling (CITC)	HIV testing initiated by the client through voluntary counselling and testing.	Stand-alone testing & counselling Mobile testing & counselling Workplace testing & counselling School testing & counselling Home-based testing & counselling Couples testing & counselling HIV self–testing
Provider–initiated Testing &Counselling	HIV testing initiated by the care provider, but where the client has the right not to be tested, through 'Opt-inn' or 'Opt-out' approach. 'Opt-in' – describes that a client must affirmatively agree to be tested. 'Opt-out' – describes that testing will continue unless the client declines to be tested.	Clinical settings PMTC Couples testing & counselling
Diagnostic HIV testing	Indicated to aid clinical diagnosis and management, including patients with HIV-related signs and symptoms, including all tuberculosis patients as part of routine management.	Clinical settings
Mandatory HIV testing screening	Mandatory screening for HIV and other blood-borne viruses of all blood donors.	Clinical settings

urce: WHO, 2009

1.4 HIVST delivery model

HIVST was first considered over 20 years ago but has had limited formal implementation in health or alternative settings. HIVST is defined as "the process whereby an individual, who is willing to know his/her HIV status collects their specimen (blood or oral fluid), performs HIV testing using a rapid diagnostic test and interprets the test results in private" (WHO 2016). The World Health Organization (WHO) recommends HIVST as a complementary approach to HTS (WHO 2016). In July 2017, WHO prequalified OraQuick HIV Self-test (OraSure Technologies Inc.) (WHO 2017), and a blood-based HIV self-test in 2018 (WHO 2018). The HIVST does not provide a definitive diagnosis but rather acts as a screening test for the presence of HIV –1/2 antibodies or HIV 1 p24 antigen (Holm-Hansen et al., 2007, WHO 2016).

Oral fluid compared with blood has a lower HIV antibody concentration; hence, slightly higher false-negative rates than blood-based tests. A reactive self–test, therefore, requires further confirmation according to relevant national testing algorithms (Ng et al., 2012, WHO 2016). An individual or a couple can either perform HIVST using home sample collection kits or home self–testing. The procedure requires users to collects a sample (e.g. oral fluid from the mouth or blood spot from a finger prick), runs the rapid test and reads the result at home either without supervision or at a health facility under the supervision of a trained care provider. Users receive pre–and post-test instructions in the information booklets contained in the test kits (Pai et al., 2013, WHO 2016).

There is documented evidence that HIVST has the potential to empower non–testers, who are mostly at high–risk, to know their HIV status (Wong et al., 2014, WHO 2016). HIVST has the potential to circumvent most facility-based barriers currently deterring individuals from testing. Previous studies have documented high acceptability of HIVST among different most–at-risk populations ranging from 70.5% among health care workers (HCWs) in Ethiopia, (Kebede et al., 2013) to 92% among serodiscordant couples in Malawi (Choko et al., 2011).

Factors associated with high acceptability of HIVST include perceived high confidentiality and privacy as well as high preference for rapid oral fluid tests compared to blood-based testing (Spielberg et al., 2000, WHO 2016).

In 2014, the OraQuick® in-home HIV self-test kit with a sensitivity of 92% and specificity of 99%, was approved by the United States Food and Drug Administration (US Food and Drug Administration (FDA) 2012, WHO 2014). Ever since, products for HIVST have increased significantly globally and currently, most commercially available HIVST rapid diagnostic tests use whole blood-based (e.g. finger pricks or capillary) or oral–fluid-based tests (UNAIDS 2013, WHO 2016, UNAIDS 2018). Most available RDTs for self-testing is easy to use, with clear instructions-for-use (IFU) in local languages and interpretation for optimized accuracy, which is understandable at low literacy and education levels (Indravudh et al., 2018).

The International Medical Device Regulation Forum classifies HIVST kits as in vitro diagnostic (IVD), which refers to test on specimens taken from the human body and considered as medical devices (Peck et al., 2014). Currently, most rapid diagnostic tests for HIVST are derived from products for professional use in assisted testing environments, for example, by modifying the labelling packaging and/or instructions. Several HIV self-test prototypes (including both oral and finger stick tests) are reported in the literature (Peck et al., 2014, (WHO). 2015, Tonen-Wolyec et al., 2018).

For example, Tonen et al. (Tonen-Wolyec et al., 2018) conducted a study among adults in the Democratic Republic of Congo to evaluate the practicability of HIVST using the prototype Exacto® Test HIV (Biosynex) self-test kits.

The Exacto® Test HIV (Biosynex) self-test consists of a bag with a test cassette, diluent vial, disinfectant wipe, compression swab, lancet, sampler stick, dressing and instruction for use. A drop of blood from a finger-prick collected by a sampler stick is placed into a SQUARE well BLOOD of the test cassette.

Two drops of diluent are shed in the ROUND well DILUENT of the test cassette for 10 minutes before reading the results (Tonen-Wolyec et al., 2018).

The Ora Quick® rapid HIV 1/2 antibody test (OraSure Technologies, Bethlehem, PA, USA) is the first WHO prequalified HIVST kit (Wong et al., 2019). The Ora Quick® rapid HIV 1/2 antibody test is a lateral-flow, immuno-chromatographic, second-generation, oral-fluid assay detecting antibodies to HIV-1 and HIV-2. The OraQuick test kits consist of two pouches; one contains a diluent tube and the second contains the test device and instruction for use.

An oral fluid swab collected using the flat-pad of the test device from upper and lower gums is placed into a pre-filled tube of reagent for 20 minutes before reading the results. The test should not be read after 40 minutes (OraSure Technologies, Bethlehem, PA, USA).

The delivery of HIVST services can be categorized into two approaches. The first approach describes the access to HIVST, which can be clinically restricted, semi-restricted or non-restricted. Clinically restricted access refers to when health care professionals provide HIV self-test kits as per national guidelines or policy. Semi-restricted is when health workers or volunteers provide support in terms of pre-test instructions and counselling before distributing the HIVST kits to clients (e.g., community health workers distribution). Non-restricted is when HIV self-test kits are made available through different distribution outlets, such as the use of vending machines, pharmacies, clinics, etc. (WHO 2016).

The second approach describes the distribution and initiation of HIVST, which can take place in range of places. Private HIV self-testing involves distributing HIVST kits from over the counter pharmacies, or grocery stores. Community-based HIVST involves the distribution of HIVST test kits to clients through community health workers.

Finally, supervised HIVST involves support from a health care worker who is physically present throughout the self-testing process. The amount of support provided to the user and the mode of administration or distribution of the self-test kits differentiates the two approaches.(WHO 2016). See Figure 1.1.

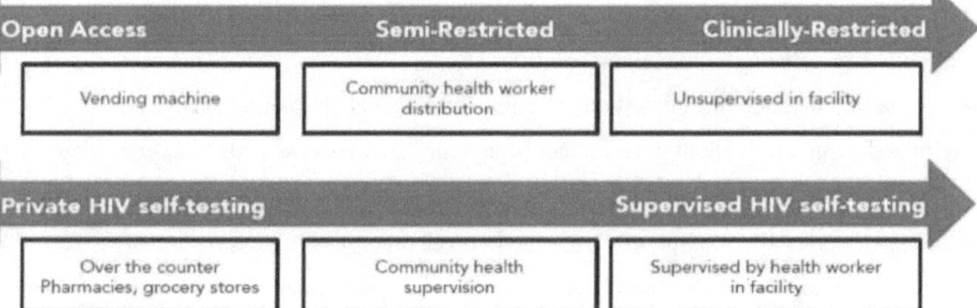

Figure 1.1. Continuums for access to HIV self-testing and distribution and initiation of HIV self-testing.

1.5 Theoretical and empirical literature

In this book, we elicit the target population intentions and context-specific factors, which may facilitate HIVST uptake through the implementation of a theory-based behaviour change intervention (BCI). The IBM was the theoretical perspective of the BCI aiming to identify factors, which may influence HIVST uptake at the individual level by stating that an individual's intentions are linked with multiple behavioural factors, which motivate individuals to undertake a recommended behaviour (e.g. HIV testing).

1.5.1 Theories of behaviour and behaviour change theories

Health behaviour for HIV risk reduction, prevention and AIDS care is a complex behaviour influenced by multi-level factors, including the individual's knowledge, attitudes, emotions and risk perceptions. Other factors include gender power dynamics in partnerships, accessibility of HTS, economic disparities, stigma and discrimination of key populations and vulnerable groups and lack of policies (Kaufman et al., 2014).

Theoretical understanding of behaviour and behaviour change is imperative to maximize the potential effects of behaviour change interventions (BCIs). Behaviour change theories signify the accrued knowledge of the methods of action and agents of change, as well as the pre-determined assumption about what human behaviour is (Davis et al., 2015).

Behaviour change theories aim to explain why behaviours change by citing interpersonal, environmental, personal and behavioural characteristics as fundamental factors in influencing behaviours. There is an increased interest in the application of behaviour change theories in health-related areas, including HIV (Kaufman et al., 2014, Deuba et al., 2020).

There is a distinction between models of behaviour and theories of change, whereby models are diagnostic in nature, specifically used in understanding the psychological factors that explain or forecast a specific behaviour (Glanz et al., 2008). Theories, on the other hand, are process-oriented and aim at changing specific behaviour. Hence, from the behaviour change viewpoint, understanding behaviour and changing behaviour are two distinct but complementary parts of behaviour change research (Glanz et al., 2008). Most individual-level behavioural theories have been widely used in BCI for HIV-related behaviours, with varying behavioural outcomes (Kaufman et al., 2014, Deuba et al., 2020).

Currently, BCIs tend to adopt theories that address individual or/and interpersonal rather than social and environmental variables (Glanz et al., 2008). Kaufman et al. argue for a shift from individual-level or interpersonal-level interventions to multi-level approaches to HIV-related behaviour change (Kaufman et al., 2014). The multi-level approaches include using formative studies to select appropriate levels and context-specific variables; measuring social and institutional variables at a proper level to ensure significant assessments of multiple levels are made and the use of theoretical models and implementation frameworks to develop BCI and methods to facilitate transferability, sustainability and scalability (Kaufman et al., 2014).

1.5.2 Integrated Behavior Model (IBM)

In this book, the IBM theory was used to identify attitudes (instrumental and experiential), perceived norms (injunctive and descriptive) and personal agency (perceived control and self–efficacy), (Glanz et al., 2008) among FBWs and MCPs, to inform the design, development and evaluation of a BCI to increase HIVST uptake and linkage to HIV prevention, care and treatment.

Besides, IBM helps to identify factors, which motivate individuals to undertake a recommended behaviour (e.g. HIVST). The theory is also useful to identify factors that need to be addressed to change behaviour and is composed of three key constructs, which are (a) attitude towards the behaviour; (b) perceived norms; and (c) personal agency (Baranowski et al., 2002, Bandura 2006).

According to the IBM, a person's attitude towards a behaviour refers to an individual's emotional reactions towards performing the behaviour and their beliefs about the anticipated positive or negative consequences related to the recommended behaviour. The concept of "perceived norms" refers to perceived social pressure from significant others to perform or not perform a behaviour. The concept of "personal agency" refers to the individual's ability to engage in the behaviour (Bandura 2006).

The theory postulates that attitudes can be experiential or instrumental. Fishbein refers to an experiential or affects attitude as a person's emotional reaction to the idea of performing the behaviour. He argues that a negative or positive emotional reaction may influence an individual's willingness to perform a behaviour. Further, individuals with a strong negative emotional reaction are less likely to perform the behaviour than individuals with a strong positive emotional reaction (Fishbein 2007). An instrumental attitude, on the other hand, is cognitive in nature and influenced by underlying beliefs about the anticipated positive or negative consequences related to the recommended behaviour (Fishbein 2007).

The implication for BCI is that providing information about potential benefits of behaviour (for example HIVST) and correcting misconceptions about potential negative consequences may increase the likelihood of intending to perform the behaviour.

According to Baranowski (2002), an "injunctive norm" refers to an individual's belief about the extent to which other people who are important to them think they should or should not perform a particular behavior (Baranowski et al., 2002). The concept of "descriptive norms" refers to an individual's perception of what his or her peers or significant others do regarding the behaviour. Both injunctive and descriptive norms are important components of normative influence in social identity in most cultures (Bagozzi and Lee 2002). For example, if a FBW believes that a relative (e.g. her mother) expects her to undertake an HIV self–test then it is more likely that she will perform a self–test. On the other hand, if a FBW perceives that her mother would undergo HIVST, this will influence her decision to accept the self–testing. The implication for a behavioural change intervention is that uncovering injunctive and descriptive norms that support a behaviour will positively influence a person's intention to perform the behaviour.

The concept of "personal agency" includes two theoretical constructs: "self–efficacy" and "perceived control". "Self–efficacy" is the confidence an individual has in his or her capacity to perform the desired behaviour.

"Perceived control" refers to an individual's perceived likelihood of occurrence of each facilitating or constraining condition and beliefs about the effect of facilitators and barriers on behavioural performance. The individual's ability to perform the required task and the influence of various environmental factors may determine the degree of perceived control. Baranowski, et al. hypothesize that perceived control influences behaviour directly and through intention (Baranowski et al., 2002, Bandura 2006, Glanz et al., 2008).

For example, knowledge about how and where to access HIVST, availability of the test kit and constraints such as lack of transport, the cost of testing or long waiting times to access the test kit might influence a person's sense of agency concerning HIVST. See Figure 1.2. below.

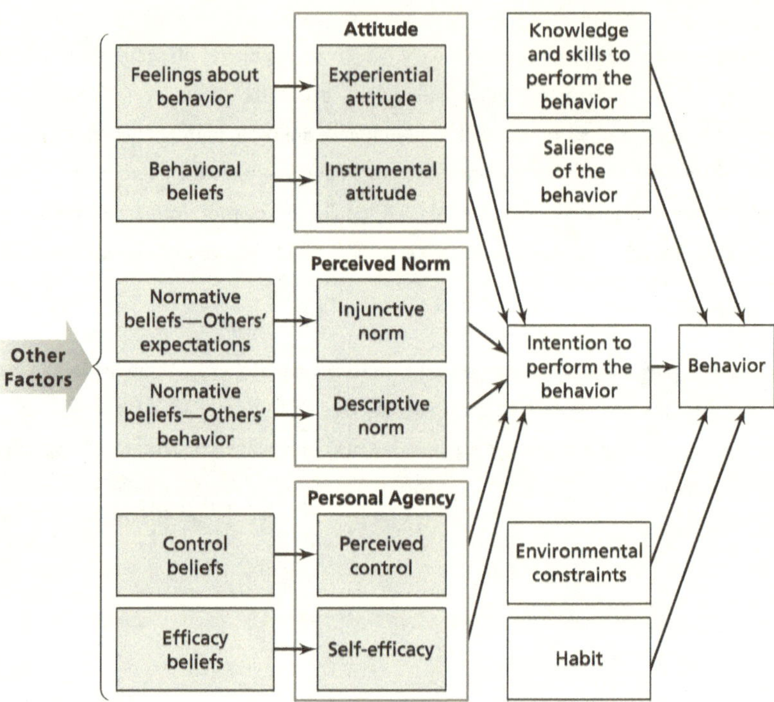

Figure 1.2. The Integrated Behavior Model (adapted from Glanz et al., 2008).

1.5.3 The PRECEDE-PROCEED Model

In this book, the PRECEDE-PROCEED model was adopted as a road map to provide a structure for applying theories and implementation frameworks systematically to plan and evaluate a behaviour change intervention.(Green and Kreuter 1999).

The PRECEDE-PROCEED model is a cost-benefit evaluation framework, which can assist health planners, interventionists and policymakers to conduct situational analysis and efficiently develop health interventions (Green and Kreuter 1999).

The PRECEDE-PROCEED model is a comprehensive planning and evaluation guide made up of two key concepts: PROCEED refers to predisposing, reinforcing and enabling constructs in educational diagnosis and evaluation and PROCEED refers to policy, regulatory and organizational constructs in educational and environmental development (Glanz et al., 2008).

The model has strong theoretical and practical foundations and assist interventionists to plan effective BCI by using behaviour change theories. Unlike behaviour change theories, the purpose of the model is not to predict or describe the relationship of variables influencing outcomes of interest (Glanz et al., 2008).

According to Green and Kreuter, the model's trademark methods include: flexibility and scalability, evidence-based process and outcome evaluations, the principle of participation and process for appropriate adaptation of evidence (Green and Kreuter 1999).

Further, the PRECEDE-PROCEED model allows the application of intrapersonal theories of health behaviour although the model is social-ecological in nature. The social-ecological nature of the model emphasizes the impact of social, cultural, economic and environmental factors on the population health (Green and Kreuter 1999). The model is population-centred incorporating behaviour change theories focusing on population health rather than individuals (Green and Kreuter 2005). However, Green and Kreuter (2005) noted that: "people learn continuously from their environmental and social surroundings and can develop, individually or collectively, the knowledge and skills to modify them" (Green and Kreuter 2005). This observation emphasises considering the use of individual theories constructs, such as personal agency from the Social Cognitive theory to achieve a democratic social behaviour change (Bandura 2004).

Like the implementation frameworks, which commence as a progression of stages to follow to have an adequate process of implementation, the PRECEDE-PROCEED model moves through the layers of a social-ecological model starting from individual characteristics to the broad socio-political environment, underlining the full participation of the 'target population' in every phase of the model (Green and Kreuter 2005). This concurs with the argument that human behaviour is complex and influenced by multiple factors. Hence, understanding the context in which they occur and the associated social factors are crucial for developing and evaluating an effective BCI (Davis et al., 2015).

The PRECEDE-PROCEED model suggests that health behaviour is influenced by a wide span of predisposing, enabling and reinforcing factors. According to the model, great consideration should be invested in this range of factors during the designing of the health promotion intervention (Green and Kreuter 1999). The PRECEDE-PROCEED planning model involves four planning phases, one implementation phase and three evaluation phases. Evidence suggests the successful application of the model in a wide range of settings, to guide the design, development, implementation and evaluation of the BCIs (Mokdad et al., 2004).

The model postulates that health promotion interventions could be created as a diagnostic approach, commencing with the final quality of life goal and finishing with the health promotion intervention i.e., direct attention to outcomes and not inputs (Green and Kreuter 1999).

The framework starts with desired outcomes, and works retrospectively in the causal chain to determine a combination of strategies for gaining the specified objectives (Glanz et al., 2008). Active participation of the target population in defining their health problems, setting their goals and developing their solution is a fundamental supposition of the model (Green and Kreuter 1999). Table 1.2. summarizes the phases of the PRECEDE-PROCEED model.

Table 1.2. Phases of the PRECEDE-PROCEED planning model	
PRECEDE phases	**PROCEED phases**
Phase 1- Social Diagnosis	Phase 5-Implementation
Phase 2- Epidemiological, Behavioural & Environmental Diagnosis	Phase 6-Process Evaluation
Phase 3-Educational & Ecological Diagnosis	Phase 7-Impact Evaluation
Phase 4-Administrative & Policy Diagnosis	Phase 8- Outcome Evaluation
Adapted from Glanz et al., (2008).	

1.5.4 Key phases of the PRECEDE-PROCEED planning model

The PRECEDE-PROCEED model is divided into six phases, which provide step-by-step guidance on intervention development and aspects for intervention evaluation. (Green and Kreuter 1999, Glanz et al., 2008).

Phase 1 of the PRECEDE-PROCEED planning model begins with a social assessment-referred as " the application, through broad participation, of multiple sources of information, both objective and subjective, designed to expand the mutual understanding of people regarding their aspirations for common good" (Glanz et al., 2008). The social assessment includes a review of the relevant scientific literature and theory for planners to expand their understanding of the health problem from the target population.

Phase 2 of the PRECEDE-PROCEED model identifies and priorities health issues and set change objectives. In this phase, the model identifies structural barriers to health by assessing the physical, social, political and environmental determinants. The epidemiological analysis helps planners to identify the health problems, concerns or goals on which the intervention would address. Besides, this process exposes the behavioural and environmental factors most probable to affect the identified priority health problems. Finally, this investigation assists to convert those priorities into measurable objectives for the development of the intervention (Glanz et al., 2008). Planners should adopt behavioural change theories and determine how the theory constructs can assist to stipulate behavioural and environmental factors, which influence the health problem of interest identified in phase 1 above.

Phase 3 of the PRECEDE-PROCEED model begins with planners evaluating the broader causal factors behind the social and health issues prioritized in phases 1 and 2. In assessing the causal factors, the model incorporates different constructs from intrapersonal theories. Examples of the intrapersonal theories include the Health Belief Model (Rosenstock 1990), Social Cognitive Theory (Bandura 1977, Bandura 2004), Theory of Reasoned Action (Fishbein and Azjen 1975) and initial stages of the Transtheoretical Model (Glanz et al., 2008). The causal factors are divided into three categories: *Predisposing factors*, which include individual knowledge and attitudes, based on the intrapersonal theories. *Enabling factors* include the resources and skills needed for the decision-making process to achieve desired behavioural and environmental changes.

Concepts such as social capital, community capacity and collective efficacy play a crucial role in identifying the enabling factors. *Reinforcing factors* are those providing the external rewards or incentives including positive (or negative) feedback for the continuation of a behaviour. The intrapersonal theories described above are very helpful in this part of the model.

Planners should priorities all three categories of factors, identify behaviour change techniques (BCTs) that may be effective in bringing about behavioural change and decide on practical strategies to put the BCTs into action.

Phase 4 of the PRECEDE-PROCEED model focuses on the alignment of the components of the intervention, intervention functions and the BCTs identified in phase 3 above. Planners should look at two levels (i.e., macro and micro levels) during the alignment process. At the macro level, planners should consider the organizational and environmental systems that affect environmental change. At the micro-level, planners focus on 'best strategies' that could directly influence the target population's behaviour change.

Phase 5 of the PRECEDE-PROCEED model deals with the implementation and evaluation of the intervention. Planners should have data collection plans in place for evaluating the process and outcome of the intervention. Process evaluation determines the extent to which the intervention was implemented as planned. Outcome evaluation determines the impact of the intervention on intended health behaviour indicators. The goal is to make the intervention available, accessible, acceptable and accountable. Besides, the intervention should be practically feasible, appropriate to the needs, desires and context of the 'target population'.

Table 1.3. below shows the six key phases of the PRECEDE-PROCEED model adopted as a 'road map' in this book. The conceptualization of the PRECEDE-PROCEED model is described in detail in **Chapter Six**.

Table 1.3. PRECEDE-PROCEED model for the development and implementation of behaviour change intervention.

Sub –study objectives	The PRECEDE-PROCEED phases
Sub-study 1: Addressing book objective 1: To systematically review the evidence on the effects of HIVST on the uptake of testing, the yield of new HIV positive diagnosis, social harms and linkage to ART treatment and barriers to and facilitators for HIVST among adults in Africa.	Phase 1: Identifying the evidence-practice gap on HIVT uptake. A systematic review and qualitative evidence synthesis identifying the evidence-practice gap on HIVST uptake.
Sub-study 2: Addressing book objective 2: To explore perceptions of key informants, community members and the target population in Northern Tanzania, and contextual and organizational factors related to HIVST to inform the development of the behaviour change intervention.	Phase 2& 3: Identifying behavioral/or environmental determinants. Educational and ecological assessment. A formative study addressing key informant's understanding about the motivation and beliefs of the community towards HIVST and target population's attitudes, beliefs and personal agency towards HIVST uptake.

Sub-study 2: Addressing book objectives 1 & 2 as described above.	Phase 4: Development of the BCI. Design and development of a theory-based behaviour change intervention to increase HIVST uptake, linkage to HIV prevention, care and treatment.
Sub-study 2: Addressing book objective 3: To evaluate the acceptability, feasibility and fidelity of the behaviour change intervention among FBWs and MCPs.	Phase 5: Implementation and evaluation of the BCI. Implementation of a theory-based behaviour change intervention and process and outcome evaluation accessing targets the population's beliefs, attitudes and personal agency to increase HIVST uptake and linkage to HIV prevention, care and treatment.
Sub-study 2: Addressing book objective 4: To evaluate the impact of the behaviour change intervention on FBWs and MCPs beliefs, attitudes and personal agency to increase HIVST uptake and linkage to HIV prevention, care and treatment.	

Table 1.3. PRECEDE-PROCEED model for the development and implementation of the behaviour change intervention *(Adapted from Watson,* et al., 1999).

1.6 Implementation strategies

Implementation strategies are defined as " an integrated set, bundle, or package of discreet implementation interventions ideally selected to address specific identified barriers to implementation success" (Proctor et al., 2013). Implementation strategies are complex and can vary widely. For example, BCIs may use a single component strategy e.g. counselling guidelines to change counsellor's behaviour. These are also known as discrete strategies or "implementation interventions'.

In the implementation of science literature, there exists a list and taxonomies that highlights the range of these strategies (Powell et al., 2012, Mazza et al., 2013, Michie et al., 2013, Proctor et al., 2013). For instance, Michie et al. have published a taxonomy of 93 behaviour change techniques, which could be used to modify specific implementation strategies for BCIs (Michie et al., 2013). Frequently, combinations of strategies form a multi-level intervention, which includes training, consultation, audits and feedback.

Whether using discrete or multi-level strategies, it is imperative to specify the strategy by first naming or labelling, giving a conceptual definition and operationalization (by defining the 'actor', 'the action' and 'action target', temporality or sequence, dose or intensity, affected implementation outcome and justification). Implementation strategies are complex social interventions since they tackle multifaceted and complicated mechanisms within interpersonal, organizational and social contexts. Hence, the complexity of the implementation strategies presents one of the greatest challenges to their distinct description, functional definition and measurement (Proctor et al., 2013). To circumvent the above-mentioned challenge, Proctor et al (2013) described several pre-requisites to the measurement of implementation strategies. They emphasised the importance of naming or labelling an implementation strategy using language that is similar to current implementation science literature. They argue that this step will circumvent the problems of using multiple meanings for the same term(s), different terms with similar or coinciding meanings and random changes in the previously mentioned. Interventionists should take considerable measures to name implementation strategies by using commonly used terminologies in implementation science literature. According to Proctor et al (2013), the naming of implementation strategies may become a challenge when designing a multi-level intervention using a wide range of separate implementation strategies. Hence, interventionists should make every effort to specify the separate components of the implementation strategies (Proctor et al., 2013).

The second step is to define the implementation strategy grounded on theoretical frameworks. Such a definition provides a broader overview of what the strategy may involve and allows for a distinct comparison of whether the terminologies are similar or not with terms used in the existing implementation literature. This applies also to complex multi-level implementation strategies whereby each of the discrete strategies are differentiated and defined conceptually (Proctor et al., 2013).

The next important step is the operationalization of the implementation strategies. This step ensures the application of the strategies in the way they were pre-determined during the development of the BCI.

This step is very important when assessing the fidelity of implementation by demonstrating the delivery strategy according to plan. According to Proctor et al. (2013), there are seven dimensions, which constitute adequate operationalization of implementation strategies.

The seven dimensions are: (a) the actor(s)-those who deliver the strategies (trained peer-educators); (b) the action-reflects the implementation efforts, feedback, support and proposed changes over time (fidelity of implementation) (c) the target(s)-those newly trained on the innovation (FBWs and MCPs). Other dimensions are (d) temporality- the order or phase of implementation (PRECEDE-PROCEED model); (e) dosage-at what frequency and intensity (fidelity of implementation); (f) the implementation outcome(s) affected-the uptake of the innovation among target users, the fidelity of implementation and sustainability of the innovation; and justification- supported by theoretical, empirical, or pragmatic justification (Proctor et al., 2013).

In this book Michie's taxonomy of 93 behaviour change techniques (Michie et al., 2013), was used to identify and operationalise the implementation strategies used in the theory-based BCI described in **Chapter Six**.

1.6.1 Implementation outcomes

Conceptualization and evaluation of successful BCIs is a critical concern in implementation research. The universal lack of implementation outcomes in reported theory-based BCIs is widely reported in implementation science literature (Rosen and Proctor 1981, Proctor et al., 2011, Proctor et al., 2013). According to Rosen and Proctor (1981), implementation outcomes are defined as "the effects of deliberate and purposive actions to implement new treatments, practices and services".

Implementation outcomes are made up of three key functions namely (a) indicators of the implementation success, (b) proximal indicators of process and (c) key intermediate outcomes concerning service system or clinical outcomes in treatment effectiveness and quality of care research (Rosen and Proctor 1981). Implementation outcomes are prerequisites for achieving consequent anticipated changes in service outcomes, to have effective BCI. There are three types of outcomes in implementation research as presented in a conceptual framework by Proctor et al (2013). In his conceptual framework, Proctor et al. (2013), distinguish between three distinct, but interrelated types of outcomes (a) implementation, (b) service, (c) client outcomes as shown in Figure 1.3.

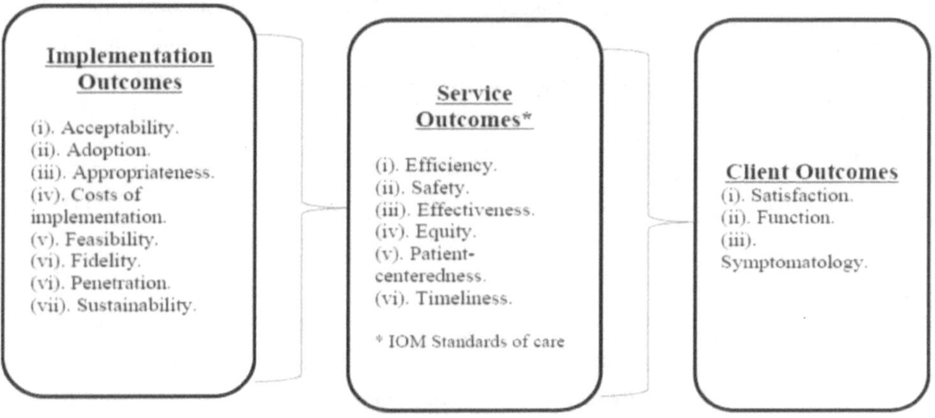

Figure 1.3. Types of outcomes in implementation research (Source: Proctor et al., 2011).

In brief, implementation outcomes include seven components, namely (a) acceptability, (b) adoption, (c) appropriateness, (d) implementation costs, (e) feasibility, (f) fidelity, (g) penetration and (h) sustainability. Service outcomes include six components, namely (a) efficiency, (b) safety, (c) effectiveness, (d) equity, (e) patient-centeredness and (f) timeliness. Client outcomes include three components, namely (a) satisfaction, (b) function, and (c) symptomatology.

Proctor et al. (2013) argue that implementation research requires conceptually and empirically distinct from those of service and clinical effectiveness, hence implementation outcomes precede both service and client outcomes (Proctor et al., 2013).

Acceptability as an implementation outcome refers to implementer's perception that an innovation (e.g. HIVST) is agreeable, palatable, or satisfactory within a particular setting. The assumption is that acceptability is dynamic, changing with experience and hence may change along the implementation continuum. *Adoption* of "uptake" is the intention, initials decision, or action taken to initiate an innovation (e.g. HIVST). *Appropriateness* refers to the perception that a specific innovation (e.g. HIVST) is fit, relevant, or compatible for a given setting, implementers, or users. Besides, "appropriateness" refers to the perceived fit of a specific innovation to address a particular health problem. "Appropriateness" can be regarded as being similar to "acceptability".

Proctor et al. (2011), argue that there is a distinction between the two terms. Innovation can be perceived as appropriate but not acceptable and vice versa (Proctor et al., 2011). *Implementation cost* refers to the cost-effectiveness of an implementation effort.

Three components determine the true cost of implementing an innovation. These are the cost of the specific intervention, the implementation strategies used and the setting of service delivery. *Feasibility* refers to the extent to which innovation is utilised or implemented within a given setting. This underscores the importance of including stakeholder interviews presented in **Chapter Five**. *Fidelity* refers to the extent of innovation implementation following a pre-defined protocol or implementer's desired intention. Five dimensions measure fidelity of implementation. These include (a) adherence (i.e. the degree to which intervention is delivered as per protocol), (b) exposure to the intervention (i.e. number and lengths of sessions implemented, frequency of implementation techniques) and (c) quality of delivery (i.e. ways in which an intervention is delivered). Other dimensions are (a) participants' responsiveness (i.e. the extent to which participants are involved in the content of an intervention) and (b) recruitment strategy (i.e. the procedures that are used to get eligible participants).

Penetration refers to the integration of innovation within service settings and relevant sub-systems and *Sustainability* is defined as the degree to which a newly implemented innovation is maintained or scaled-up within functional service settings (Proctor et al., 2011). For this book, implementation outcomes namely "acceptability", "feasibility" "uptake" and "fidelity " were adopted and described more in **Chapter Six.**

In summary, a discussion of theories, which are essential to behaviour change approaches and its constructs are applied widely to modify individual, social and environmental factors that determine health behaviour. In combination, these theories have assisted interventionist to avoid simplistic suppositions, such as raising awareness and providing health education on a health problem, such as HIV and focus on mechanisms for behaviour change.

These theories, which underline social cognitive viewpoints of behaviour, are important because of their ability to illuminate processes underpinning individual behaviour and help to identify methods of change and guidance in the development of effective BCIs. However, existing evidence suggests that constructs from these theories account for a moderate percentage of variance in behaviour. Thus, a focus on the theories is imperative, but with limitations.

The key to understanding individual behaviour and intentions to change lies within the relevant economical, physical and social environment. An interventionist must put into consideration the influence of environmental factors on motivation, intentions, skills and behaviour for effective BCIs. Using a single theory or model in the development and evaluation of a BCI in a real-life environment is usually inadequate or inappropriate. To overcome this impediment, it is to use integrated theories, which combine variables from theories such as the HBM, TRA, TPB, SCT, etc.
The rationale for selecting the PRECEDE-PROCEED model lies in the fact that it is a community-based and participatory framework in nature.

The model was considered suitable for this project because it emphasizes the active participation of target populations (in this book, the FBWs and MCPs who intend to participate in the BCI) in the planning process. The framework highlights the importance of including end-users in the implementation process, which is of relevance in this project. The framework can be used to repetitively assimilate planning and evaluation stages, assist priorities setting and resource allocation, and provide a mechanism to guide intervention activities. The model permits the establishment of variables important in evaluating the BCI because the desired outcomes are defined at the beginning of the planning phases. The PRECEDE-PROCEED model could be used to facilitate the transferability of the processes of BCI to comparable environments and at different levels in the community.

The main limitation of the PRECEDE-PROCEED model, however, is the lack of guidance available related to the PROCEED evaluation phases, despite the recommendation to link particular evaluative phases to specific PRECEDE phases (Green and Kreuter 2005).

1.7 Literature review

The objectives of the literature review were to (a) identify existing evidence on the potential of HIVST to increase HIV testing and linkage to HIV prevention care and treatment (b) identify evidence on the usefulness of the Integrated Behavior Model (IBM) in developing and evaluating testing interventions and (c) identify needs for further research. To synthesize evidence on the usefulness of IBM on uptake of and feasibility of HIVST, a literature review was conducted in PubMed using the keywords: IBM, HIV, AIDS, HIVST, Uptake, Adults and Africa. Both acronyms and actual full search terms were used. Studies were identified that met the following criteria (a) included behavioural theory models (i.e. IBM); (b) considered uptake of HIV testing as a dependent variable of interest; and c) were conducted in Africa.

The literature review focused on existing evidence of HIV self–testing strategies and the extent to which they increased uptake of HIV testing and linkage to HIV prevention, care and treatment by reaching key populations in different settings.

There is evidence that HIVST has the potential to empower non–testers who are high–risk, to know their HIV status in privacy (Johnson et al., 2014).Three systematic reviews, all conducted in 2013 provide evidence on HIV self–testing globally, including SSA. Pai, et al. (2013) performed a systematic review on supervised (self–testing and counselling aided by a health care professional) and unsupervised (performed by self–tester with access to phone/internet counselling) self–testing strategies among high and low-risk populations (Pai et al., 2013). Krause, et al. (2013) conducted a systematic review on the acceptability of HIV self–testing in high– and low–income countries. Suthar, et al. (2013) conducted a systematic review and meta-analysis to seek evidence for the community–based HTS; including self–testing (Suthar et al., 2013).

The Pai, et al. review included 21 studies of which, two–thirds evaluated oral self–testing and a third evaluated blood self–testing. Seven (7) and fourteen (14) studies evaluated unsupervised and supervised HIVST respectively. Seventeen studies (89%) came from high–income settings and only four (11%) studies were from Africa (Malawi n = 3; Kenya n.=.1). Lastly, the study subjects varied from most–at–risk of HIV infection to low–at-risk general populations. The main objectives of the review were to evaluate the current evidence on the implementation of supervised and unsupervised HIV self-test strategies. Specifically, the review outcomes were acceptability, accuracy, feasibility, cost and post-test counselling. Additionally, synthesis was done on information on challenges, concerns and barriers derived from qualitative or mixed-method studies (Pai et al., 2013).

Eleven studies were included in Krause, et al. review. Nine were conducted in high–income countries while two were from Africa (Malawi n = 1; Kenya n = 1). The review objectives included acceptability, review of the accuracy of HIVST, linkage to care of new HIV–positives, disclosure of self–testers, utilisation of telephone hotlines for counselling and qualitative attributes of HIVST.

The study subjects were heterogeneous key population groups including health care workers (HCWs), men having sex with men (MSM), people who inject drugs (PWIDs) and/ or people who use drugs (PWUDs), as well as clients of sexual transmitted infection (STI) clinics, women with multiple sexual partners or HIV seropositive sexual partners and the general population.

In less than a fifth (18.2%) of the studies were the samples collected at home. Out of 11 studies, one (9.1%) evaluated blood-based and oral fluid-based rapid tests, two (18.2%), evaluated blood-based and eight (72.7%) evaluated oral–fluid-based rapid tests. Finally, most of the data were from observational studies (82 %) and only two intervention studies (Krause et al., 2013).

The Suthar, et al. (2013) review included 117 studies, reported on HIVST self–testing. The review outcomes were the uptake of HTS, first–time testers, CD4 count for HIV–positives, HIV–positivity rate, coverage, HIV incidence and cost per person tested. The study subjects were from the general population including key populations such as MSM and PWIDs/ PWUDs (Suthar et al., 2013).

1.7.1 Acceptability and uptake of HIVST

Pai, et al. (2013), defined acceptability as the number of people who self–tested divided by the number who consented to self–test for both supervised and unsupervised testing strategies and reported high acceptability ranging from 74% to 96% (Pai et al., 2013).

Seven studies using supervised strategies reported acceptability ranged from 74% in MSM in the US to 24% in HIV clinic attendees in the US. For unsupervised strategies, acceptability in two studies ranged from 22% among HCWs in Kenya to 84% among MSM in the United States of America. There was also evidence for a higher preference for HIV self–testing compared to facility-based testing and oral-based rather than blood-based self–testing (Pai et al., 2013).

The review concurs with Krause, et al. (2013) findings on high acceptability on HIVST among the majority of participants. Krause, et al. defined acceptability as the proportion of all people approached to participate in a study that eventually performed HIVST (Krause et al., 2013). Of the 10 studies included, the acceptability ranged from 22% to 87.2%. The highest acceptability (87.2%) was in a study done in Malawi among sero discordant couples in the home-based unsupervised self–testing.

Interestingly, in this study acceptability was similar for both genders despite a low testing history among men. However, a study in Kenya among HCWs reported a low acceptance rate of 21.9%. The key reason for the low acceptability was the low–attendance at pre-testing sessions where self–test kits were distributed in public (Krause et al., 2013).

A meta-analysis comparing different community–based HTS approaches by Suthar, et al. (2013) reported participant's high uptake of self–testing compared with school-based HTS, with a pooled estimate of 86.9% of participants doing self–testing compared with 62% doing school-based HTS. The review defined uptake – instead of acceptability – as the proportion of participants accepting HTS over those offered HTS (Suthar et al., 2013).

1.7.2 Feasibility and accuracy of HIVST

The feasibility of HIVST is a major concern particularly concerning linkage to HIV prevention, care and treatment. Ten studies included in Pai, et al. (2013) review measured the feasibility of self–testing with different outcomes across the studies.

The review defined feasibility as documentation of completion of the self–testing and counselling process. Overall, a certain pattern of testing errors was observed. Documented errors in test performance included (a) incorrect placement of the oral test device after swabbing, (b) early removal of the test device from the developer (c) poor handling of the developer fluid and (d) immersing the test device in the developer solution without swabbing the gums.

However, one unsupervised study found about 95% of MSM reported that the kits were "very easy to use", with no testing user errors (Pai et al., 2013).

The accuracy of self-test kits is another key concern related to HIVST among laypersons, HIV policymakers and implementers. The Krause, et al. (2013) review reported high accuracy among subjects in performing HIV self–testing.

Seven out of 11 studies measured the accuracy i.e. the proportion of self–test results in agreement with confirmatory test results performed and interpreted by trained health staff (Krause et al., 2013). The concordance in test results between laypersons and health care providers in a supervised self–testing strategy was 86%. Out of the seven studies, the highest concordance was 99% of valid test results in a Spanish study. In Singapore, the discordance of test results was 54% and was due to the incorrect transfer of a blood sample with a capillary tube. Misinterpretation of very faint lines in the self–tests and unknown HIV–positive status was associated with invalid test results. The omission of demonstrations of testing procedures by trained health staff may also explain performance errors (Krause et al., 2013).

Pai, et al. (2013) observed differentials in the measurements of accuracy between supervised and unsupervised self– testing. Four (one unsupervised, three supervised) out of 21 studies measured specificity and sensitivity of self– tests. The specificity of self–tests, i.e. the chance of an HIV–negative person receiving a negative test result, in both strategies was high (range: 74%–96%), while the sensitivity, i.e. the chance of an HIV–positive person receiving a positive test result, was lower in the unsupervised subjects (range: 92.9% –100%) than supervised (range: 97.4%– 97.9%). Slightly lower sensitivity of 92.9% was reported in high–prevalence settings (HIV > 1%), compared to a sensitivity of 100%, in low–prevalence settings (HIV < 1%). This observation raises a key concern of the possibility of misclassification of an HIV–positive person as HIV negative in unsupervised self–testing strategies (Pai et al., 2013).

1.7.3 Barriers, motivators and preferences to HIVST

Apart from the common barriers associated with uptake of HTS in general, there are additional barriers related to HIVST. The knowledge gaps about HIVST, lack of both policies and regulatory systems, ethical and human rights concerns are an example of barriers reported in the literature (Johnson et al., 2014). In 2014, according to Wong, et al. only five countries, the USA, France, UK, Kenya and Zambia reported having national policies related to HIVST (Wong et al., 2014).

However, recent evidence on HIVST reported that 59 countries are having, or developing national policies in a global acceleration towards the expansion of HIVST access for increased diagnostic coverage (Wong et al., 2019).

The misperception about the inaccuracy of self-test kits is another key barrier to scaling–up of HIVST. For example, a qualitative study to explore preferences of different HIV testing approaches among potential clients in Tanzania showed uncertainty on perceptions of the accuracy of HIV self–test kits and regarded self–testing as the least feasible option (Njau et al., 2014). However, several studies have documented the high accuracy and acceptability of oral fluid rapid HIV testing (Holm-Hansen et al., 1993, Campbell and Klein 2006, Wright and Katz 2006, Holm-Hansen et al., 2007, Xun et al., 2013).

For potential users who fear needle pricks for obtaining a blood sample may find blood-based HIVST testing a barrier. The oral fluid HIV rapid diagnostic tests are the more preferred option because they are simpler, user-friendly and less invasive (Xun et al., 2013).

Another barrier is the cost of buying the self-test kits. Most people in low and middle-income countries (LMICs), including African countries, may not afford to pay for the self-test kits, which range from $ 4.8 to $ 40 in different settings (Johnson et al., 2014). However, most governments in low–income countries either do not recommend or do not financially support HIVST.

Some studies report that respondents suggested that free rapid oral fluids HIV self–test kits should be available through government subsidies (Choko et al., 2011). High–priced oral fluid HIV rapid testing affects scale–up efforts in most LMICs, including in SSA (Johnson et al., 2014).

Finally, the inability to read among potential users may limit the uptake of unsupervised HIVST, whereby an individual is supposed to test following the instruction for use document while testing alone in privacy.

However, a supervised self–testing strategy, which includes the use of local language, demonstration of self– testing procedures by trained counsellors, accompanied with a video or leaflets using graphic instructions may circumvent this barrier (Choko et al., 2011).

The Pai, et al. (2013) review documented several motivators for HIVST of which key were (a) convenience (b) short and quick testing time(c) privacy (d) autonomy/sense of empowerment and (e) perceived control of one's health choices. Also, the review reported a high preference for rapid oral fluid tests compared to blood-based testing. This may indicate a preference for a simple, less–invasive procedure, compared with needle pricks used to draw blood samples. Other advantages of oral fluid HIV tests are easy to sample collection and acquisition, a minimum waiting time of 20 minutes before getting a result, reduction of needle injuries, low viral load in oral fluids and safer waste materials disposal (Pai et al., 2013).

1.7.4 Linkage to HIV prevention, care and treatment

Linkage to HIV prevention, care and treatment is the ultimate goal for making people in the general population aware of their HIV status. All three reviews discussed above reported lack of evidence about linkage to post-test counselling, prevention, treatment and care services among those who tested HIV positive using HIVST (Krause et al., 2013, Pai et al., 2013, Suthar et al., 2013).

From the evidence, it is clear that linkage–to–care will be a major self–testing implementation challenge, while maintaining privacy, which is key in self–testing strategies. Therefore, there is a need for feasibility studies on implementing HIVST to evaluate the completion of the HIV care process from testing to linkage to HIV prevention, care and treatment (Walensky and Bassett 2011).

1.7.5 Concerns and gaps related to HIVST

The literature review presents a discussion of the achievements in combating HIV pandemic globally and highlights concerns and gaps related to HIVST.

HIV policymakers and implementers have expressed concerns regarding HIVST at the individual level, HIV self–tests reliability and linkage to HIV prevention, treatment and care. One of the key concerns at the individual level is the possibility of coercion to self–test particularly among couples, which can be compounded with potential psychological harm because of the lack of post-test counselling (Carballo-Dieguez et al., 2012, Katz et al., 2012). Besides, older individuals compared to their younger counterparts may not perceive themselves at risk and therefore may not undertake self–testing. Finally, there is a concern that self–testing may encourage unprotected sexual intercourse when people know their HIV status.

In terms of the self- test, the concern is the window period – the time between suspicion of HIV infection and detection of HIV antibodies by the assay (Holm-Hansen et al., 2007). In fact, most rapid diagnostic tests have a six to 12 week window period (Holm-Hansen et al., 2007). The current cost of HIV self–test kits ranges from $0.50 to $50 and may be a drawback to the uptake of HIVST (UNAIDS 2013, UNAIDS 2018). Another concern related to the HIVST test is suspicion of adherence to the self–testing protocol. There is also concern on how to design instructions that are easy to understand and follow. An additional concern raised is the linkage to the HIV prevention and care services post-testing after HIVST (Choko et al., 2011, Mavedzenge et al., 2011). Despite all these concerns, which are valid and call for more research, currently, there is no strong evidence to show that self–testing has increased social harms or adverse effects compared with other testing modes (US Food and Drug Administration(FDA) 2012).

Innovative interventions to attract KVPs to undertake HIV testing, such as HIVST, have shown the potential to circumvent facility-based barriers to HIV testing. Facility-based barriers to HIV testing include fear of visibility, long-queues and long waiting time (UNAIDS 2019). Despite existing evidence on the potential of HIVST however, there are still gaps in the literature in LMICs about HIVST uptake and linkages to HIV prevention, care and treatment.

A 2014 study by Johnson, et al. for example, identifies key knowledge gaps in HIVST scaling–up that call for further research. The key knowledge gaps are in understanding how HIVST may change healthcare-seeking behaviours of an individual, or on how the overlap of other HIV testing services can influence the public health impact and cost-effectiveness of HIVST (Johnson et al., 2014). Lastly, there is a need to understand how the consequences may vary in different settings, the proportion of people with a positive HIVST result who receive confirmatory testing, or who are diagnosed HIV positive results and the link to treatment and care and the HIV– negative people who are linked to prevention services (Johnson et al., 2014).

Besides, systematic reviews on the acceptability of HIVST uptake reported gaps on the acceptability of unsupervised HIVST strategy, particularly in SSA. Another gap was lack of affirmative information on post-diagnosis linkage to HIV prevention, care and treatment outcomes. There was limited information on the yield of newly HIV–positive diagnoses required to increase HIV testing (Krause et al., 2013, Pai et al., 2013, Suthar et al., 2013).

References

Administration(US Food and Drug Administration(FDA))., U. F. a. D. (2012). *OraQuick In-Home HIV test summary of safety and effectiveness*. Retrieved from Silver Spring: FDA, 2012.

Allen, S., Meinzen-Derr, J., Kautzman, M., Zulu, I., Trask, S., Fideli, U. . . . Haworth, A. (2003). Sexual behaviour of HIV discordant couples after HIV counselling and testing. *AIDS, 17*(5), 733-740. Doi:10.1097/01.aids.0000050867.71999.ed

Assembly, U. N. G. (2011). *Political Declaration on HIV/AIDS: intensifying our efforts to eliminate HIV/AIDS*. Retrieved from New York, USA. http://www.unaids.org/en/media/unaids/contentassets/documents/document/2011/06/20110610_una-res-65-277_en.pdf.

Bagozzi, R. P., & Lee, K.-H. (2002). Multiple Routes for Social Influence: The Role of Compliance, Internalization and Social Identity. *Social Psychology Quarterly, 65*(3), 226. Doi: 10.2307/3090121

Bandura, A. (2006a). GUIDE FOR CONSTRUCTING SELF-EFFICACY SCALES, In A. Bandura (Ed.), *Self-Efficacy Beliefs of Adolescents* (pp. 307-337): Information Age Publishing.

Bandura, A. (2006b). Towards a Psychology of Human Agency. *Perspectives on Psychological Science. 1(2)*, 164-180.

Baranowski, T., Perry, C., & Parcel, G. (2002). How individuals, environments and health behaviour interact: Social Cognitive Theory. In K. Glanz, B. Rimer & F. M. Lewis (Eds.), Health Behaviour and Health Education: Theory, research and practice (3rd ed., pp. 165-184). San Francisco: Jossey-Bass.

Bateganya, M. H., Abdulwadud, O. A., & Kiene, S. M. (2008). Home-based HIV voluntary counselling and testing in developing countries. *Cochrane Database of Systematic Reviews* (4), 1-32. Doi:10.1002/14651858.CD006493.pub2

Campbell, S., & Klein, R. (2006). Home testing to detect human immunodeficiency virus: boob or bane? *Journal of Clinical Microbiology, 44*(Critical Appraisal Skills Programme 2010), 3473-3476. Doi:10.1128/JCM.01511-06.

Carballo-Dieguez, A., Balan, I., Frasca, T., Dolezal, C., & Valladares, J. (2012). *Use of a rapid HIV home test to screen potential sexual partner prevents HIV exposure in a high-risk sample of MSM.* Washington (D.C.). http://pag.aids2012.org/abstarcts.aspx?aid=4982

Carballo-Dieguez, A., Frasca, T., Dolezal, C., & Balan, I. (2012). Will gay and bisexually active men at high risk of infection use over-the-counter rapid HIV test to screen sexual partners? *Journal of Sex Research, 49*, 379-387. Retrieved from http://www.tandfonline.com/Doi/pdf/10.1080/00224499.2011.647117

Choko, A. T., Desmond, N., Webb, E. L., Chavula, K., Napierala-Mavedzenge, S., Gaydos, C. A. . . . Corbett, E. L. (2011). The uptake and accuracy of oral kits for HIV self-testing in high HIV prevalence setting a cross-sectional feasibility study in Blantyre, Malawi. *PLoS Medicine, 8*(Critical Appraisal Skills Programme 2010), e1001102. Doi:10.1371/journal.pmed.1001102

Corbett, E. L., Daya, E., Matambo, R., Cheung, Y. B., Makamure, B., Bassett, and M. T. . . . Hayes, R. J. (2006). Uptake of workplace HIV counselling and testing: a cluster-randomized trial in Zimbabwe. *PLoS Medicine, 3*(7), e238. Doi:10.1371/journal.pmed.0030238

Critical Appraisal Skills Programme 2010. (Critical Appraisal Skills Programme 2010). Critical Appraisal Skills Programme (CASP). 10 questions to help you make sense of qualitative research. England: Critical Appraisals Skills Programme 2010. Retrieved from http://www.casp-uk.net/wp-content/uploads/2011/11/CASP Qualitative Appraisal Checklist 14oct10.pdf.

Fishbein, M. (2007). A Reasoned Action Approach: Some Issues, Questions and Clarifications. In I. Ajzen, D.Albaraccin, & R.Hornik. (Eds.), *Prediction and Change of Health Behaviour: Applying the Reasoned Action Approach.* Hillsdale, N.J.: Erlbaum, 2007.

Gardner, L. I., Metsch, L. R. Anderson-Mahoney, P., Loughlin, A. M., del Rio, C., Strathdee, S., . . . Access Study Study, G. (2005). Efficacy of a briefcase management intervention to link recently diagnosed HIV-infected persons to care. *AIDS, 19*(4), 423-431. Retrieved from http://www.ncbi.nlm.nih.gov/pubmed/15750396

http://graphics.tx.ovid.com/ovftpdfs/FPDDNCLBNBFBLN00/fs047/ovft/live/gv031/00002030/00002030-200503040-00008.pdf

Glanz, K., Rimer, B. K., & Viswanath, K. (2008). *Health behaviour and health education: theory, research and practice* (4th Ed.). San Francisco: Jossey-Bass.

Govindasamy, D., Kranzer, K., van Schaik, N., Noubary, F., Wood, R., Walensky, R. P. . . . Bekker, L. G. (2013). Linkage to HIV, TB and non-communicable disease care from a mobile testing unit in Cape Town, South Africa. *PLoS ONE, 8*(11), e80017. Doi:10.1371/journal.pone.0080017

Holm-Hansen, C., Constatine, N. T., & Hukenes, G. (1993). Detection of antibodies to HIV in homologous sets of plasma, urine and oral mucosal transudate samples using rapid assays in Tanzania. *Clinical Diagnostics & Virology, 1*, 207-214.

Holm-Hansen, C., Nyombi, B., & Nyindo, M. (2007). Saliva-based HIV Testing among Secondary School Students in Tanzania using the OraQuick Rapid HIV 1/2 Antibody Assay. *Annals of New York Academic of Sciences, 1098*, 461-466.

Hutchinson, A. B., Branson, B. M., Kim, A., & Farnham, P. G. (2006). A meta-analysis of the effectiveness of alternative HIV counselling and testing methods to increase knowledge of HIV status. *AIDS, 20*(12), 1597-1604. Doi:10.1097/01.aids.0000238405.93249.16

Johnson, C., Baggaley, R., Forsythe, S., van Rooyen, H., Ford, N., Napierala Mavedzenge, S., . . . Taegtmeyer, M. (2014). Realizing the Potential for HIV Self-Testing. *AIDS Behaviour*. Doi: 10.1007/s10461-014-0832

Kalibala, S., Tun, W., Cherutich, P., Nganga, A., Oweya, E., & Oluoch, P. (2014). Factors associated with acceptability of HIV self-testing among health care workers in Kenya. *AIDS Behaviour, 18 Suppl 4*, S405-414. Doi: 10.1007/s10461-014-0830-z.

Kalichman, S. C., Cherry, C., Amaral, C., White, D., Kalichman, M. O., Pope, H., . . . Macy, R. (Critical Appraisal Skills Programme 2010). Health and Treatment Implications of Food Insufficiency among People Living with HIV/AIDS, Atlanta, Georgia. *Journal of Urban Health: Bulletin of the New York Academy of Medicine, Vol. 87, No. 4*. Doi: 10.1007/s11524-010-9446-4

Katz, D., Golden, M., Hughes, J., Farquhar, C., & Stekler, J. (2012). *Acceptability and ease of use of Home self-testing for HIV among MSM*. Paper presented at the 19th Conference on Retroviruses and Opportunistic Infections, Seattle (Washington).

Kebede, B., Abate, T., & Mekonnen, D. (2013). HIV self-testing practices among Health care Workers: feasibility and options for accelerating HIV testing services in Ethiopia. *Pan African Medical Journal, 15*(50), 1-8.

Kranzer, K., Govindasamy, D., van Schaik, N., Thebus, E., Davies, N., Zimmermann, M. . . . Bekker, L. G. (2012). Incentivized recruitment of a population sample to mobile HIV testing services increases the yield of newly diagnosed cases, including those in need of antiretroviral therapy. *HIV Medicine, 13*(2), 132-137. Retrieved from http://onlinelibrary.wiley.com/store/10.1111/j.1468-1293.2011.00947.x/asset/hiv947.pdf?v=1&t=i64uvopm&s=eff3584783d70d2d1cf6624b0d94291fbbd23aaf

Krause, J., Subklew-Sehume, F., Kenyon, C., & Colebunders, R. (2013). Acceptability of HIV self-testing: a systematic literature review. *BMC Public Health, 13* :(735.), 1-19.

Kumwenda, M., Munthali, A., Phiri, M., Mwale, D., Guttenberg, T., MacPherson, E. . . . Desmond, N. (2014). Factors shaping initial decision-making to self-test amongst cohabiting couples in urban Blantyre, Malawi. *AIDS Behaviour, 18 Suppl 4*, S396-404. Doi: 10.1007/s10461-014-0817-9

MacPherson, P., Webb, E. L., Choko, A. T., Desmond, N., & Chavula, K., et al. (2011). Stigmatizing attitudes among people offered home-based HIV testing and counselling in Blantyre, Malawi: construction and analysis of a stigma scale. *PLoS One 6: e26814*. Doi:*10.1371/journal.pone.0026814*.

Mavedzenge, S. N., Baggaley, R., Lo, Y. R., & Corbett, L. (2011). HIV self-testing among health workers: a review of the literature and discussion of current practices, issues and options for increasing access to HIV testing in Sub-Saharan Africa.

Menzies, N., Abang, B., Wanyenze, R., Nuwaha, F., Mugisha, B., Coutinho, A. . . . Blandford, J. M. (Effective Practice and Organisation of Care 2009). The costs and effectiveness of four HIV counselling and testing strategies in Uganda. *AIDS, 23*, 395-401. Retrieved from http://graphics.tx.ovid.com/ovftpdfs/FPDDNCLBABCDJD00/fs047/ovft/live/gv024/00002030/00002030-200901280-00014.pdf

Morin, S. F., Khumalo-Sakutukwa, G., Charlebois, E. D., Routh, J., Fritz, K., & Lane, T. (2006). Removing barriers to knowing HIV status: same-day mobile HIV testing in Zimbabwe. *Journal of Acquired Immune Deficiency Syndromes, 41*(2), 218-224. Retrieved from http://graphics.tx.ovid.com/ovftpdfs/FPDDNCLBABCDJD00/fs047/ovft/live/gv031/00126334/00126334-200602010-00014.pdf

Naik, R., Doherty, T., Jackson, D., Tabana, H., Swanevelder, S., Thea, D. M. . . . Fox, M. P. (2015). Linkage to care following a home-based HIV counselling and testing intervention in rural South Africa. *Journal of International AIDS Society, 18*(19843).

Ng, O. T., Chow, A. L., Lee, V. J., Chen, M. I. C., Win, M. K., Tan, H. H., . . . Leo, Y. S. (2012). Accuracy and User-Acceptability of HIV Self-Testing Using an Oral fluid-based HIV Rapid Test. *PLoS ONE 7(Effective Practice and Organisation of Care 2009): e45168.* Doi:*10.1371/journal.pone.0045168.*

Njau, B., Ostermann, J., Brown, D., Mühlbacher, A., Reddy, E., & Thielman, N. (2014). HIV testing preferences in Tanzania: a qualitative exploration of the importance of confidentiality, accessibility and quality of service. *BMC Public Health, 14*, 838-847. Doi: 10.1186/1471-2458-14-838

Njau, B., Watt, M. H., Ostermann, J., Manongi, R., & Sikkema, K. J. (2012). Perceived acceptability of home-based couples voluntary HIV counselling and testing in Northern Tanzania. *AIDS Care, 24*(4), 413-419. Doi:10.1080/09540121.2011.608796

Obermeyer, C. M., & Osborn, M. (2007). The Utilization of Testing and Counselling for HIV: A Review of the Social and Behavioural Evidence. *American Journal of Public Health, 97*(Critical Appraisal Skills Programme 2010), 1762-1774. Doi: 10.2105? AJPH.2006.096263

The organization, W. H. (2013). *Consolidated guidelines on the use of antiretroviral drugs for treating and preventing HIV infection: recommendations for public health approach.* Retrieved from http://www.who.int/hiv/pub/guidelines/arv2013/.

WHO (2014). *March 2014 supplement to the consolidated guidelines on the use of antiretroviral drugs for treating and preventing HIV infection, recommendations for a public health approach. Consolidated.* Retrieved from Geneva:

Ostermann, J., Njau, B., Brown, D. S., Muhlbacher, A., & Thielman, N. (2014). Heterogeneous HIV testing preferences in an urban setting in Tanzania: results from a discrete choice experiment. *PLoS ONE, 9*(3), e92100. Doi:10.1371/journal.pone.0092100

Pai, N. P., Behlim, T., Abrahams, L., Vadnais, C., Shivkumar, S., Pillay, S. . . . Dhenda, K. (2013). Will an Unsupervised Self-testing Strategy for HIV work in health Care Workers of South Africa? A Cross-Sectional Pilot Feasibility Study. *PLoS ONE, 8*(11), e79772.

Pai, N. P., Sharma, J., Shivkumar, S., Pillay, S., Vadnais, C., Joseph, L. . . . Peeling, R. W. (2013). Supervised and Unsupervised Self-Testing for HIV in High- and Low-Risk Populations: A Systematic Review. *PLoS Medicine, 10(4):* e1001414.

Peck, R. B., Lim, J. M., van Rooyen, H., Mukoma, W., Chepuka, L., Bansal, P. . . . Taegtmeyer, M. (2014). What should the ideal HIV self-test look like? A usability study of test prototypes in unsupervised HIV self-testing in Kenya, Malawi and South Africa. *AIDS Behaviour, 18 Suppl 4*, S422-432. Doi: 10.1007/s10461-014-0818-8

Poobalan, A. S., Pitchforth, E., Imamura, M., Tucker, J. S., Philip, K., Spratte, J. . . . van Teijlingeng, E. (Effective Practice and Organisation of Care 2009). Characteristics of effective interventions in improving young people's sexual health: a review of reviews. *Sex Education.9: 3, 319–336.* Doi: 10.1080/14681810903059185

Spielberg, F., Critchlow, C., Vittinghoff, E., Coletti, A. S., Sheppard, H., Mayer, K. H. . . . Gross, M. (2000). Home collection for frequent HIV testing: acceptability of oral fluids, dried blood spots and telephone results. HIV Early Detection Study Group. *AIDS, 14*(12), 1819-1828. Retrieved fromhttp://www.ncbi.nlm.nih.gov/pubmed/10985320http://graphics.tx.ovid.com/ovftpdfs/FPDDNCGCGBGHBD00/fs035/ovft/live/gv010/00002030/00002030-200008180-00018.pdf.

Suthar, A. B., Ford, N., Bachanas , P. J., Wong, V. J., Rajan, J. S., Saltzman, A. K., . . . Baggaley, R. C. (2013). Towards Universal Voluntary HIV Testing and Counselling A Systematic Review and Meta-Analysis of Community-Based Approaches. *PLoS Medicine, 10(8) :*(e1001496.). Doi:10.1371/journal.pmed.1001496

Sweat, M., et al. (2000). The Voluntary HIV-1 Counselling and Testing Efficacy Study: A Randomized Controlled Trial in Three Countries. Retrieved from www.ingentaconnect.com/content/klu/aibe/2000

Sweat, M., Morin, S., Celentano, D., Mulawa, M., Singh, B., Mbwambo, J. . . . Team: P. A. S. (2012). Community-based intervention to increase HIV testing and case detection in people aged 16-32 years in Tanzania, Zimbabwe and Thailand (NIMH Project Accept, HPTN043). *Lancet Infectious Diseases, 11*, 525-532.

Sweat, M., Morin, S., Celentano, D., Mulawa, M., Singh, B., Mbwambo, J. . . . Team, a. t. P. A. S. (2011). Increases in HIV Testing and Case Detection from NIMH Project Accept (HPTN 043) among 16–32-Year-Olds: A Randomized Community-Based Intervention in Tanzania, Zimbabwe and Thailand. *Lancet Infectious Diseases, 11*(7), 525–532.

Tonen-Wolyec, S., Batina-Agasa, S., Muwonga, J., Fwamba N'kulu, F., Mboumba Bouassa, R. S., & Belec, L. (2018). Evaluation of the practicability and virological performance of finger-stick whole blood HIV self-testing in French-speaking sub-Saharan Africa. *PLoS ONE, 13*(1), e0189475. Doi:10.1371/journal.pone.0189475

UNAIDS. (2013). *Global report: UNAIDS report on the global AIDS epidemic 2013.In.Geneva, Switzerland.* Retrieved from

UNAIDS. (2014). *A short Technical Update on Self-Testing for HIV.* Retrieved from

UNAIDS. (2015). *HOW AIDS CHANGED EVERYTHING: MDG 6: 15 YEARS, 15 LESSONS OF HOPE FROM THE AIDS RESPONSE.* Retrieved from

UNAIDS. (2017). UNAIDS Data

UNAIDS. (2018). *Global AIDS Update 2018: Miles To Go Closing Gaps Breaking Barriers Righting Injustices.* Retrieved from http://www.unaids.org/sites/default/files/media_asset/miles-to-go_en.pdf

UNAIDS, & WHO. (2004). *UNAIDS/WHO Policy Statement on HIV Testing.* Retrieved from

VCT. (2000). Efficacy of voluntary HIV-1 counselling and testing in individuals and couples in Kenya, Tanzania and Trinidad: a randomized trial. The Voluntary HIV-1 Counselling and Testing Efficacy Study Group. *Lancet, 356*(9224), 103-112. Doi: S0140673600024466 [pii]

Walensky, R. P., & Bassett, I. V. (2011). HIV Self-testing and the Missing Linkage. *PLoS Medicine, 8*(Critical Appraisal Skills Programme 2010), 1-2. Doi:10.1371/journal.pmed.1001101

Wanyenze, R. K., Hahn, J. A., Liechty, C. A., Ragland, K., Ronald, A., Mayanja-Kizza, H., . . . Bangsberg, D. R. (2011). Linkage to HIV care and survival following inpatient HIV counselling and testing. *AIDS Behaviour, 15*(4), 751-760. Doi: 10.1007/s10461-010-9704-1

Wanyenze, R. K., Nawavvu, C., Namale, A. S., Mayanja, B., Bunnell, R., Abang, B. . . . Kamya, M. R. (2008). Acceptability of routine HIV counselling and testing and HIV seroprevalence in Ugandan hospitals. *Bulletin of the World Health Organization, 86*, 302-309. Retrieved from http://www.ncbi.nlm.nih.gov/pmc/articles/PMC2647415/pdf/07-042580.pdf

Waters, R. C., Ostermann, J., Reeves, T. D., Masnick, M. F., & Thielman, N. M., et al. (2011). A cost-effectiveness analysis of alternative HIV re-testing strategies in sub-Saharan Africa. *Journal of Acquired Immune Deficiency Syndromes 2011, 56:443-452.*

WHO. (2008). Towards Universal Access: Scaling up Priority HIV/AIDS Interventions in the Health Sector Retrieved from http:www.who.int/hiv/pub/towards_universal_access_report_2008.pdf. Retrieved October 2009 http:www.who.int/hiv/pub/towards_universal_access_report_2008.pdf

WHO. (Effective Practice and Organisation of Care 2009). *New WHO recommendations: Preventing mother-to-child transmission.* Retrieved from

WHO. (2013a). *HIV/AIDS: Definition of key terms: consolidated ARV guidelines, June 2013*. Retrieved from www.who.int/hiv/pub/guidelines/arv2013/intro/keyterms/en/

WHO. (2013b). *Report on the first international symposium on self-testing for HIV: the legal, ethical, gender, human rights and public health implication of HIV self-testing scale-up*. Retrieved from http://apps.who.int/iris/bitstream/10665/85267/1/9789241505628_eng.pdf.

WHO. (2018). *Public Report for INSTI HIV Self-test (PQDx 0002-002-01) [Internet]*. Retrieved from https:// www.who.int/diagnostics_laboratory/evaluations/pq-list/181130_pqdx_0002_002_01_pqpr_insti_self_ test.pdf? ua=1

WHO/UNAIDS. (2007). *Guidance on Provider-initiated HIV counselling and Testing in Health facilities*. Retrieved from Geneva Switzerland:

Wong, V., Jenkins, E., Ford, N., & Ingold, H. (2019). To thine own test, be true: HIV self - testing and the global reach for the undiagnosed. *Journal of the International Aids Society, 22*(S1), e25256. Doi:10.1002/jia2.25256

Wong, V., Johnson, C., Cowan, E., Rosenthal, M., Peeling, R., Miralles, M., Brown, C. (2014). HIV Self-Testing in Resource-Limited Settings: Regulatory and Policy Considerations. *AIDS Behaviour, 18 Suppl 4*, S415-421. Doi: 10.1007/s10461-014-0825-9

(WHO). W. H. O. (2015). WHO prequalification: Sample product dossier for an IVD intended for HIV self-testing. SIMUTM self-test for HIV 12O working document, December 2015.

World Health Organization. (2016). *Guidelines on HIV self-testing and partner notification: supplement to consolidated guidelines on HIV testing services*. Retrieved from France.

World Health Organization. (2017). *WHO prequalifies first generic hepatitis C medicine and first HIV self-test. In: Essential medicines and health products [Internet]*. Retrieved from http://who.int/medicines/news/2017/1st_generic-hepC_1stHIVself-test-prequalified/en/

Wright, A. A., & Katz, I. T. (2006). Home testing for HIV. *New England Journal of Medicine, 354*(5), 437-440. Doi: 10.1056/NEJMp058302

Xun, H., Kang, D., Huang, T., Qian, Y., Li, X., Wilson, E. C. . . . Ma, W. (2013). Factors Associated with Willingness to Accept Oral Fluid HIV rapid Testing among Most-at-Risk Populations in China. *PLoS ONE, 8*(11), e80594. Retrieved from http://www.ncbi.nlm.nih.gov/pmc/articles/PMC3834295/pdf/pone.0080594.pdf

CHAPTER TWO

2.0 Overview of the project

2.1 Rationale for a theory-based behaviour change intervention (BCI)

There have been significant achievements in the fight against HIV/AIDS in Africa in general, and SSA in particular. The most recent AIDS update by UNAIDS reports that there was a 28 % decrease in new infections in SSA between 2018 and 2010 statistics (UNAIDS 2019). In 2018, there was a 44% decrease in AIDs related deaths compared to 2010 statistics (UNAIDS 2019).The uptake of HTS despite these achievements is still low however in most SSA countries with high HIV prevalence. Statistics of 2018 showed that almost 20 % of HIV–positive clients had never previously tested for HIV status in the general population (UNAIDS 2019).

In most SSA countries, nationally representative data on HIV testing shows that the overall HIV prevalence does not correlate with the uptake of testing. The overall percentage of women and men aged 15–49 who received an HIV test in the previous 12 months varies with time. Women are more likely to have tested for HIV and collected their results in the previous 12 months than their male counterparts (Staveteig et al., 2013, UNAIDS 2019).

HIV awareness is the first step in the HIV continuum of care and prevention through HTS, which is an entry point to the achievement of viral suppression. To achieve viral suppression, PLHV need to be aware of their HIV infection status, being linked and engaged in care and initiate and adhere to ART regimen (Cox et al., 2019, UNAIDS 2019).

Although global epidemiological estimates reveal downward trends in the epidemic, persistent gaps in the HIV care continuum do exist (Cox et al., 2019, UNAIDS 2019). As of 2018, about 58% of all PLHV managed to achieve viral suppression, is lower by 20 %, which is far lower than the 2020 target of 73% set by UNAIDS (UNAIDS 2019).

To achieve the target of 95–95–95 by the year 2030, effective evidence-based interventions (EBIs) to increase HTS uptake is imperative. This will only be possible by identifying appropriate EBIs (i.e. relevant for specific local settings based on the social context of target populations), which are effective and acceptable and implemented with success to provide asymptomatic positive individuals with an opportunity to know their HIV status (Cox et al., 2019). Existing evidence suggests different effective interventions to increase HTS uptake globally (UNAIDS 2019). In their review of the evidence of intervention strategies to improve men's uptake of HTS in SSA, Hlongwa et al. (2019) reported education about HIV, Community –Based HTS, Home-Based HTS, Antenatal Care HTS, HTS incentives and HIVST as effective interventions to improving HTS among men (Hlongwa et al., 2019, Hlongwa et al., 2020).

A formative study guided by the Integrated Behavior Model conducted among young men in Dar es Salaam reported high HIVST acceptability with a positive attitude and high personal agency and confirmatory HIV testing. The study recommends a peer-based intervention to promote HIVST through peer-network to address negative attitudes towards HIVST (Conserve et al., 2018).

In Northern Tanzania, FBWs and MCPs are categorized as high-risk populations and previous studies have documented the high prevalence of HIV infections (19% to 26%) among more than 1000 FBWs because of their high–risk behaviours (Kapiga et al., 2002). Many FBWs are semi-employed and may supplement their meagre salaries by providing sex services to their clients.

Thirty percent of FBWs reported receiving gifts or money in exchange for sex, while 6 % reported having had an STI through unprotected sexual intercourse. In 2015, studies conducted in Northern Tanzania estimated 17,000 MCPs between the ages of 18 and 45 years, predominantly young men who receive infrequently but sizeable payments plus extra money from tourists, spending extended time away from their spouses and engaging in multiple sexual partnerships and transactional sex (Ostermann et al., 2015, Lyamuya et al., 2017).

Besides, MCPs share many characteristics with other high HIV prevalence KVPs, such as long-distance lorry drivers, anglers, miners and migrant farm workers (Ostermann et al., 2014, Ostermann et al., 2015). A recent study among FBWs has documented that a substantial proportion (87.4 %) have been tested at least once in their lifetime, but do not re-test after engaging in high-risk behaviours for HIV infection (Njau et al., 2015). There is, however, a dearth of information regarding HIV testing/ and re-testing history among MCPs in the study setting.

Previous studies conducted in Northern Tanzania have noted that FBWs and MCPs have different preferences for HTS uptake. FBWs and MCPs showed different preferences for HTS compared to the general population. For example, FBWs preferred weekday testing, testing places where ART is available and finger pricks to oral testing compared to females in the general population. On the other hand, MCPs preferred disclosure of test results to their spouses, testing places where ART is available and finger pricks to oral testing compared to males in the general population (Ostermann et al., 2014, Ostermann et al., 2015).

Given the multi-faceted nature of factors influencing HIVST uptake including individual, social, and environmental and health system factors (as identified in the literature review presented in **Chapter One**) a behaviour change approach is imperative to address the problem of low HTS uptake among the target population.

A behaviour change approach can assist to address individual's knowledge, attitudes, beliefs and perceptions that influence the health-seeking behaviour for HIV testing among MCPs and FBWs.

Existing evidence shows that BCIs operating at an individual and population level are effective for changing HIV related risk behaviours (Lu et al., 2013, Shangani 2017, Deuba et al., 2020). For example, a review of Chinese studies reported the effectiveness of HIV- related BCI on reducing HIV risk behaviours, but not sexually infected diseases, including HIV (Lu et al., 2013). Another review on behavioural interventions to increase HIV testing among MSMs reported improvement in HIV testing as a result of peer-based interventions (Shangani 2017). Although there is strong evidence in support of the effectiveness of BCIs to reduce HIV risk behaviours in different geographical settings (Deuba et al., 2020), there is a lack of evidence on the effectiveness of population-specific as well as age-specific HIV-related BCIs for improving HIVST uptake and linkage to HIV prevention, care and treatment.

To the candidate's knowledge, in Tanzania, there are currently no studies, which have explored the acceptability and feasibility of a theory-based BCI and fidelity of implementation to increase HIVST uptake and linkage to HIV prevention, care and treatment.

To address this gap, this research developed and evaluated a theory-based BCI to increase HIVST uptake and linkage to HIV prevention, care and treatment among hard to reach adults in Northern Tanzania. The results from this intervention may provide knowledge on population-specific and age-specific theory-based BCI to increase HIVST uptake and linkage to HIV prevention, care and treatment in Northern Tanzania.

2.2 Innovation of the research

Mounting evidence demonstrates the effectiveness of ART as an HIV– prevention strategy. However, its success depends on the uptake of HIV testing and subsequent linkage to and retention in HIV care.

As described in the literature review **(Chapter One),** studies on BCIs to increase HIVST uptake are limited in African settings, including in Tanzania.

The contribution of this study is to generate information on the acceptability and feasibility of a theory-based BCI and fidelity of implementation to increase the HIVST uptake and linkage to HIV prevention, care and treatment among FBWs and MCPs in Northern Tanzania. The successful implementation of the theory-based BCI to the study target population may demonstrate the potential of an effective behaviour change approach that will be sustainable within the study settings. Finally, the study will contribute towards evidence and lay groundwork for larger studies that may compare BCIs using different theories in increasing HIVST uptake among hard to reach populations in Northern Tanzania.

2.3 Aims and objectives

This book aimed to develop and evaluate a theory-based BCI as a means of improving HIV testing coverage in hard-to-reach populations in the context of a long-standing HIV testing program. The hard to reach populations for this book were FBWs and MCPs in Northern Tanzania. This book includes four (4) objectives. Objective 1, aimed to systematically review the evidence on the effects of HIVST on uptake of HIV testing, the yield of new HIV positive diagnosis, social harms and linkage to ART treatment and barriers to and facilitators for, HIVST among adults in Africa. Objective 2 aimed to explore perceptions of key informants, community members and the target population in Northern Tanzania and contextual and organizational factors related to HIV self-testing to inform the development of the BCI. Objective 3 aimed to evaluate the acceptability and feasibility of the BCI and fidelity of implementation among FBWs and MCPs in the study setting and objective 4 aimed to evaluate the impact of the BCI on FBWs and MCPs beliefs, attitudes and personal agency to increase HIVST uptake and linkage to HIV prevention, care and treatment. The book includes two sub-studies: (a) Sub-study 1(SS1) that addressed objective 1. (b) Sub-study 2(SS 2) that addressed objectives 2 to 4.

2.4 Study population and setting

2.4.1 Moshi Municipal Council

The study area was an urban setting in Northern Tanzania with a high HIV prevalence and low HTS uptake, as reported in the Tanzania Demographic and Household Survey (DHS) of 2010. Kilimanjaro Region has a total population of 1.6 million and an average household size of 4.3 (United Republic of Tanzania 2012). The study area is on the tourist circuit, with major national parks as well as the highest mountain in Africa, Mt. Kilimanjaro. Most tourist hotels and bars are located in Northern Tanzania. According to a recent HIV prevalence report, eight regions in the country, including two in Northern Tanzania (Kilimanjaro and Arusha), witnessed an increase in prevalence, despite the overall decline in national HIV prevalence. For example, the Kilimanjaro region had an increase in HIV prevalence of 1.9% in 2011/12 (3.8%) compared with 1.9% in 2007/08. The neighbouring Arusha region reported an increase in HIV prevalence of 1.6% in 2011/12 (3.2%) compared with 1.6% in 2007/08 (United Republic of Tanzania National Bureau of Statistics and ICF 2013).

Moshi Municipal Council is among seven (7) districts in Kilimanjaro region, Northern Tanzania. The other six districts are Rombo, Mwanga, Same, Moshi, Hai and Siha District Councils. Moshi Municipal Council has an estimated population of 184,292 in 21 wards administrative unit, with an average household size of 4.0 (United Republic of Tanzania 2012). The study site has 21 facilities providing HTS, including hospitals, health centres and free-standing VCT facilities. Also, 18 HIV care and treatment centres (CTC) provide access to antiretroviral therapy (ART) within the study setting (Ostermann et al., 2014).

2.5 Ethical considerations

The research and all activities were reviewed and approved by the Kilimanjaro Christian Medical University College Ethics Committee (CREC: 884; dated: 6/1/2016), the National Institute of Medical Research in Tanzania (NIMRlHQIR.8a/Vol. IX/2454; dated: 18/4/2017) and the Health Sciences Research Ethics Committee at the University of Cape Town in South Africa (HREC REF: 737; dated: 9/11/2016). The Tanzania Food and Drugs Authority (TFDA) approved the Oral HIV kits. All eligible participants provided written consent. Participants were aware of their voluntariness to participate and the freedom to withdraw at any point from the research.

References

Bateganya, M. H., Abdulwadud, O. A., & Kiene, S. M. (2008). Home-based HIV voluntary counseling and testing in developing countries. *Cochrane Database of Systematic Reviews*(4), 1-32. Doi:10.1002/14651858.CD006493.pub2

Choko, A. T., Desmond, N., Webb, E. L., Chavula, K., Napierala-Mavedzenge, S., Gaydos, C. A., . . . Corbett, E. L. (2011). The Uptake and Accuracy of Oral Kits for HIV Self-Testing in High HIV Prevalence Setting: A Cross-Sectional Feasibility Study in Blantyre, Malawi. *PLoS Medicine, 8*(10). Doi:10.1371/journal.pmed.1001102

Coate , T. J., Richte , R., & Cacere , C. (2008). Behavioural strategies to reduce HIV transmission: how to make them work better. *Lance , 372*, 669–684. Doi:10.1016/S0140-6736(08)60886-7

Govindasamy, D., Kranzer, K., van Schaik, N., Noubary, F., Wood, R., Walensky, R. P., . . . Bekker, L. G. (2013). Linkage to HIV, TB and non-communicable disease care from a mobile testing unit in Cape Town, South Africa. *PLoS ONE, 8*(11), e80017. Doi:10.1371/journal.pone.0080017

Kapig , S. H., Sa , N. E., Sha , J. F., Renjif , B., Masseng , E. J., Kiwel , I. E., & Esse , M. (2002). HIV-1 Epidrmic Among Female Bar Workers and Hotel Workers in Northern Tanzania: Risk Factors and Opportunities for Prevention. *Journal of Acquired Immune Deficiency Syndromes, 29(4)*, 409-417.

Kranzer, K., Lawn, S. D., Meyer-Rath, G., Vassall, A., Raditlhalo, E., Govindasamy, D., . . . Bekker, L. G. (2012). Feasibility, yield, and cost of active tuberculosis case finding linked to a mobile HIV service in Cape Town, South Africa: a cross-sectional study. *PLoS Med, 9*(8), e1001281. Doi:10.1371/journal.pmed.1001281

Lyamuya, J. E., Njau, B., Damian, D. J., & Mtuy, T. (2017). Sociodemographic and Other Characteristics Associated With Behavioural Risk Factors of HIV Infection Among Male Mountain-Climbing Porters in Kilimanjaro Region, Tanzania. *East African Health Research Journal*, 1-8. Retrieved from ÂČČÆĚĐĎĎ ĔVÂZVĂĂĚÁ

NASCOP. (2008). *Guidelines for HIV Testing and Counselling in Kenya*. Retrieved from Nairobi, Kenya: ÂČČÆĚĐ ĎĎ ĔĂĂĊÁĐ XÂ ČĂ ĚÁĊĄÆĈĚ public/---ed_protect/---protrav/---ilo_aids/documents/legaldocument/wcms_127533.pdf.

Ostermann J, Whetten K, Reddy E, Pence B, Weinhold A, Itemba D, . . . Team, C. R. (2014). Treatment retention and care transitions during and after the scale-up of HIV care and treatment in Northern Tanzania. *AIDSCcare. 2014;26(11):1352-8.* Doi*: 10.1080/09540121.2014.882493.*

Ostermann, J., Njau, B., Brown, D. S., Muhlbacher, A., & Thielman, N. (2014). Heterogeneous HIV testing preferences in an urban setting in Tanzania: results from a discrete choice experiment. *PLoS ONE, 9*(3), e92100. Doi:10.1371/journal.pone.0092100

Ostermann, J., Njau, B., Mtuy, T., Brown, D. S., Muhlbacher, A., & Thielman, N. (2015). One size does not fit all: HIV testing preferences differ among high-risk groups in Northern Tanzania. *AIDS Care, 27*(5), 595-603. Doi:10.1080/09540121.2014.998612

Ostermann, J., Njau, B., Mtuy, T., Brown, D. S., Mühlbacher, A., & Thielman, N. (2015). One size does not fit all: HIV testing preferences differ among high-risk groups in Northern Tanzania. *AIDS Care: Psychological and Socio-medical Aspects of AIDS/HIV*, 1-10. Doi:10.1080/09540121.2014.998612

SAHIVSOC (2012). Joint statement on HIV testing and counslling.Retrieved from [illegible] society-news

Sharma, M., Ying, R., Tarr, G., & Barnabas, R. (2015). Systematic review and meta-analysis of community and facility-based HIV testing to address linkage to care gaps in sub-Saharan Africa. *Nature, 528*(7580), S77-85. Doi:10.1038/nature16044

Staveteg , S., Wag , S., Hwd , S. K., Bradly , S. E. K., & Nybo , E. (2013). *Demographic Patterns of HIV Testing Uptake in sub-Saharan Africa.* Retrieved from

Tanzania, U. R. o. (2013)The . *United Republic of Tanzania, Ministry of Health and Social Welfare, National AIDS Control Programme: Third Health Sector HIV and AIDS Strategic Plan(HSHSP - III) 2013-2017.* Retrieved from Prime Minister's Offcce, Da- es-Salmaam, Apri ,2014:

THIS. (2017). *TANZANIA HIV IMPACT SURVEY(THIS) 2016-2017: PRELIMINARY FINDINGS.* Retrieved from Dar-es-Salaa m,Tanzania:

UNAIDS. (2015). *HOW AIDS CHANGED EVERYTHING: MDG 6: 15 YEARS, 15 LESSONS OF HOPE FROM THE AIDS RESPONSE.* Retrieved from

United Republic of Tanzania National Bureau of Statistics, & ICF. (2013). *HIV/AIDS Malaria Indicator Survey 2011-12. In Dar es Salaa m,Tanzani a:Tanzania Commission for AIDS, ZAC, NBS, OCGS, and ICF International;2013*The .

United Republic of Tanzania, N. B. S. (2012). *2012 Tanzania Population and Housing Census* Retrieved from Dar es Salaam: [illegible]

Walensky, R. P., Wood, R., Fofana, M. O., Martinson, N. A., Losina, E., April, M. D., . . . Paltiel, A. D. (2011). The clinical impact and cost-effectiveness of routine, voluntary HIV screening in South Africa. *J Acquir Immune Defic Syndr, 56*(1), 26-35. Doi:10.1097/QAI.0b013e3181fb8f24

Walensky, R. P., Wood, R., Fofana, M. O., Marntison, N. A., & al., L. E. e. (2010). The Clinical Impact and Co-t effectiveness of Routine Voluntary HIV screening in South Africa. *Journal of Acquired ImmunD deficiency Syndromes.*

Wog , V., Johnsn , C., Cown , E., Rosenthal, M., Peeling, R., Miralles, M., . . . Brown, C. (2014). HIV Self-Testing in Resource-Limited Settings: Regulatory and Policy Considerations. *AIDS Behavior, 18 Suppl 4*, S415-421. Doi:10.1007/s10461-014-0825-9

CHAPTER THREE

3.0 The effects of HIV self-testing on the uptake of HIV testing, linkage to antiretroviral treatment and social harms among adults in Africa: A systematic review and meta-analysis

3.1 Introduction

Globally, an estimated 38.0 million people are living with HIV, with more than 2.1 million [1.9 million–2.4 million] new HIV infections and 700,000 deaths in 2018 (UNAIDS 2019). Almost fifty-five percent of the global burden of HIV is from Africa, which is the most affected region. By 2030, the UNAIDS/WHO aimed to achieve a global target of "95-95-95" whereby 95% of adults will be aware of their HIV status, 95% of HIV positive will receive sustained antiretroviral treatment (ART) and 95% of those who are on ART will achieve viral load suppression (UNAIDS 2015, UNAIDS 2019).

Regardless of considerable efforts to increase HIV testing across African countries, the coverage is still low with up to 54 % of adults unaware of their HIV status (UNAIDS 2015). The low coverage of HIV testing undermines the ability to reach the first "90" target and impedes the scaling up HIV prevention, care and treatment services. Many HIV–positive people in Africa present late for ART, because they were unaware of their status, leading to negative consequences on treatment outcomes, such as premature death (Mukolo et al., 2013, The IeDEA and ART cohort collaborations 2014).

Existing evidence suggests that HIV self -testing (HIVST) provides an opportunity for people who do not know their HIV status and fear visiting health facilities to test for HIV (Johnson et al., 2014).

HIVST refers to a procedure whereby an individual or a couple who are willing to know their HIV status collect a specimen, perform the test and interpret the test results in private. HIVST can be classified into two categories, namely: directly assisted (supervised) or unassisted (unsupervised) HIV self–testing (UNAIDS/WHO 2004).

Directly assisted HIVST is a process whereas a user self-test for HIV under the supervision of a trained provider or peers. The support includes the manufacturer – supplied written instructions and a demonstration on how to perform a self-test and how to interpret the results. Unassisted HIVST refers to when a user self-test for HIV without supervision, but by using a self-test kit together with the manufacturer-supplied written instructions found inside the kits (UNAIDS/WHO 2004).

HIV policymakers raised several concerns regarding the introduction of HIVST across different settings globally (Lee et al., 2007, Wong et al., 2014, Sharma 2015). However, irrespective of HIV policymakers' reservations, some African countries have introduced HIVST. For example, Kenya in 2009 (NASCOP 2008), Zambia in 2011 (Wong et al., 2014), and South Africa in 2017 (SAHIVSOC 2012), have incorporated an HIVST delivery model into the national HIV testing services (HTS) policy. Furthermore, countries such as Malawi (Choko et al., 2011) and Zimbabwe (Wong et al., 2014), are considering including HIVST in policy and practice. For example, in South Africa, self-test kits are now available over the counter (SAHIVSOC 2012). Currently, 15 SSA countries have HIVST policies in place or under development (Wong et al., 2019). Most of the multi-country public evidence, which informed WHO HIVST guidelines, resulted from a five-year (2015-2020), Unitaid-funded HIV Self-testing Africa (STAR) initiative supporting HIVST in Malawi, Zambia, South Africa, Lesotho and Swaziland (STAR 2015). The aim of the initiative was to generate evidence related to the feasibility and acceptability of HIVST in Malawi, Zambia and Zimbabwe in the first two-year phase.

Lesotho, Eswatini and South Africa were added in the second three-year phase, aiming to create a market for HIVST and evaluate optimal distribution approaches for non-testers, non-repeat tester or hard to reach people (STAR 2015, Wong et al., 2019).

This systematic review aims to synthesize the evidence on the effects of HIVST among adults in Africa on the uptake of testing, the yield of new HIV–positive diagnoses, linkage to ARV treatment and the incidence of social harms.

3.2 Methods

This systematic review followed guidance from the Cochrane Collaboration (Higgins and Green 2005) and is reported based on the Preferred Reporting Items for Systematic Reviews and meta-analyses (PRISMA) statement. A review protocol was developed and registered in the PROSPERO International Prospective Register of systematic reviews: registration number: CRD42015023935) (Njau et al., 2016).

3.2.1 Eligibility criteria

Inclusion and exclusion criteria

All experimental studies, which included RCTs, before-after studies, interrupted time-series studies, and compared HIVST with a standard of HTS and/or which compared different approaches to HIVST were eligible for inclusion. We excluded editorials, reviews, perspectives and studies not assessing HIVST (e.g. home-based but non-self–test). We also excluded studies, which did not clearly define the type of HIV testing approaches. Abstracts were included if full-texts were not available. Reviewers held meetings to discuss any disagreements in the study inclusion and /or exclusion criterion and resolved them by consensus.

3.2.2 Study designs

Experimental studies including randomized controlled trials (RCTs), before-after studies and interrupted time-series studies were eligible for inclusion in this review.

3.2.3 Participants

The study participants were adults (males and females) from African countries.

3.2.4 Intervention and comparisons

A trained health care provider or a peer can deliver on how to use the HIVST self-test kits under supervision, or without supervision in privacy using manufacturer –supplied written instructions. In this review, we compared the effects of HIV self-testing, either alone, or in addition to the standard HIV testing services (HTS). Standard HTS include: (a) provider-administered testing (b) door-to-door testing (c) mobile testing (d) index testing (e) workplace testing and (f) client-initiated testing, or any combination of these approaches. We also compared different approaches to HIVST.

3.2.5 Outcomes

The primary outcomes were uptake of HIV testing and the yield of new HIV-positive diagnoses among adults in African countries. The primary outcomes were defined as:

- Uptake: the proportion of participants offered HIV testing who underwent HIV testing (Fylkenes and Siziya 2004).
-
- The yield of new HIV–positive diagnoses: the proportion of participants offered HIV testing who were newly diagnosed as HIV-positive (Walensky et al., 2002, Walensky et al., 2010).

The secondary outcomes were defined as:

- HIV positivity: the proportion of participants offered HIV testing who were diagnosed HIV positive (MacPherson et al., 2014).
- Linkage to ART: the proportion of diagnosed HIV-positive participants who were enrolled in ART at any time after testing.
- CD4 count: the proportion of diagnosed HIV-positive participants who had their CD4 count measured (Govindasamy et al., 2013).

- Social harm: the number of participants for whom any episode of harm was observed or reported, during or after HIV testing e.g. intimate partner violence, coercive testing by a partner, suicide etc. (Choko et al., 2015).

3.2.6 Setting

We included studies conducted in any country on the African continent.

3.3 Information sources

3.3.1 Electronic databases

A comprehensive search strategy was developed to identify both published and unpublished articles with no language restrictions from 1998 to 2018. All searches were conducted within the publication date limits of 1998 or the closest date limit available, reflecting the time since the emergence of advanced developments of rapid HIV diagnostic tests including self–testing (WHO 1998). The review searched for related studies in PubMed, The Cochrane Central Register of Controlled Trials (CENTRAL), Pan African Clinical Trials Registry and The Cochrane Database of Systematic Reviews (CDSR), Databases of Abstracts of Reviews of Effectiveness (DARE), Social Sciences Citation Index, Web of Science and African Index Medicus. We also searched websites and databases for grey materials such as greynet.org, World Health Organization Library Information System (WHOLIS), WHO Global Index Medicus, The Joint United Nations Programme on HIV/AIDS (UNAIDS resource library), Alliance of Health Policy & Systems Research, The World Bank. Additionally, we searched for conference abstracts from the following conference databases: International AIDS conference, 1st International symposium on self-testing for HIV, International AIDS Society Conference (IAS) and Conference on Retroviruses and Opportunistic Infections (CROI). To overcome the limitations of search functions, we used terms for self-testing to search for HIV-related conference abstracts published from 2001-2018. We also searched the HIV Self-Testing Research and Policy Hub (HIVST.org) for ongoing updates of ongoing trials.

The search strategies for electronic databases incorporated medical subject headings (MeSH), free–text terms and a comprehensive African search filter that was adapted to suit each database using an applicable controlled vocabulary (Eisinga et al., 2007, Piennar et al., 2011). Furthermore, we checked reference lists of the included studies and other relevant systematic reviews for further eligible reports using Google Scholar and Web of Science.

3.3.2 Search strategy

During the search we used various medical subject headings (MeSH) and search terms adapted to various databases such as: " adult", "young adults", "middle-aged", " aged", "aged, 80 and over", 'uptake of care", "yield", "HIV prevalence", "HIV Seroprevalence", "HIV positivity", "social harm", "HIV linkage", "linkage to care", " randomized controlled trial", "controlled clinical trial", "placebo", "HIV". Other search terms were "Human Immunodeficiency Virus", "AIDS", "Acquired Immunodeficiency Syndrome", counsel*, test*, HIV test*, "HIV self-testing", "unsupervised self-testing", "supervised self-testing", "provider-administered testing", "randomized controlled trial," 'clinical trials as a topic," "randomly", "trial', Africa*, South* AND Africa*, North* AND Africa*, East* AND Africa*, Central* AND Africa*, SUB SAHARAN AFRICA* SUB SAHARAN AFRICA*. Searches were combined with the names of each country in Eastern, Northern and Southern Africa by using the Boolean operators "OR" or "AND". The search was restricted to human subjects. The full search string for PubMed is included in the appendix. We sought expert views on the search strategy to assess the search terms proposed for this review (Appendix A).

3.4 Study records

3.4.1 Data management

We merged all search results into a reference management software EndNote and removed duplicate records of the same report.

3.4.2 Selection process

Two authors (BN and DD) screened the search outputs to select potentially eligible studies. BN then obtained the full text of potentially eligible studies and then both authors (BN and DD) conducted the final study selection for inclusion in the review independently. We used a PRISMA flow chart to summarize the search and selection of studies for the review as shown in Table 3.1.

3.4.3 Data collection process

Two reviewers (BN and DD) independently extracted data using a pre-designed data extraction form (Appendix B). A third reviewer (LA) was available to solve any differences of views between the two reviewers that arose. A pilot trial of the data extraction form was conducted to check its adequacy and necessary changes were made.

3.4.4 Data items

Extracted data included study design, study settings or place (e.g. city/ country/or rural/urban or facility-based /community–based), year of study, year of publication (i.e., 1998 to 2018), type of HIVST approaches (e.g. direct assisted or unassisted), type of comparator (e.g. standard HIV testing services), study population (e.g. general population or key populations) and study outcomes of interest.

3.5 Assessment of risk of bias in included studies

Two authors (BN and DD) independently assessed the risk of bias (low risk of bias, high risk of bias, or unclear risk of bias) using the Cochrane risk of bias instrument. The risk of bias assessment includes an assessment of sequence generation and allocation concealment (selection bias), blinding of participants and personnel (performance bias), blinding of outcome assessment (detection bias), incomplete outcome data (attrition bias), selective reporting (reporting bias) and unclear risk of bias (either due to lack of information or uncertainty over the potential bias). The two reviewers resolve any disagreements between them by consensus. Trials reporting > 20 percentage of missing data were assessed at a high risk of attrition bias.

Because of the nature of HIV testing studies, blinding of participants and/or researchers to the interventions is difficult, giving way to the potential of introducing bias. The reviewer was cautious to judge the methodological quality of the trails as poor, but rather acknowledged the possibility of performance or detection biases. The assessments of risk of bias are summarized in tables 3.1-3.3 and figure 3.6.

3.6 Investigation of heterogeneity

We used the I^2 statistics to evaluate the heterogeneity of results for each outcome, across trials. Values of 25, 50 and 75 % were interpreted as a low, medium and high heterogeneity respectively.

3.7 Assessment of reporting biases

To reduce publication bias we applied search strategies to include relevant unpublished studies. We searched the grey literature, including conference proceedings (e.g., International AIDS Conference) and prospective trial registration databases to over-come time-lag bias. A funnel plot is indicated to investigate publication bias if there were ≥ 10 trials included in analysis.

The aim was to determine the likelihood of smaller studies to exaggerate the magnitude of effects. However, this review did not use a funnel plot test because of fewer trials (n=5), where the power of tests is too low to distinguish chance from publication bias.

3.8 Data analysis

For outcomes with more than ≥ 2 trials available, we pooled intervention effect estimates using the random-effects model design. We reported the estimate of the effects as risk ratios with corresponding 95% confidence intervals (CI) for each outcome included in the review. Where researchers reporting on cluster-randomized trial data as if randomization was performed at an individual level rather than the cluster, we requested from the leading author for the intra-cluster correlation coefficient (ICC).

We planned to use the ICC to reanalyze the trial data to obtain approximate correct analyses according to the description in the Cochrane Handbook for Systematic Reviews of Interventions. However, none of the selected cluster RCTs reported randomization at the individual level (Review Manager [RevMan] 2014).

3.9 Sensitivity analysis

We planned to conduct sensitivity analysis to: (a) evaluate the effect of excluding studies unable to meet each quality criterion affect the overall estimate and (b) evaluate the change in the results if only high-quality studies where included. We also planned to conduct a sensitivity analysis to assess the potential bias that may have occurred because of the inadequately controlled clustered trials. However, the sensitivity analysis was not done to evaluate the prediction interval and present the range of effects because of the small number (n=5) of trials included in this review (Borenstein et al., 2017).

3.10 Results

Two thousand six hundred and seventeen (2,617) citations were identified through electronic search and other sources, which after screening resulted in five RCTs (two individually randomized trials and three cluster-randomized) meeting the review eligibility criteria (Figure 3.1). There are ongoing RCT conducted by The Self-Testing (STAR) Initiative in Malawi (NCT02718274; NCT 03541382; NCT03271307; ISRCTN 18421340), Zimbabwe (NCT 03559959), Lesotho, Zambia (NCT02793804), Uganda (NCT 02846402) and Kenya (NCT03135067).

3.10.1 Study characteristics

Five RCTs (MacPherson et al., 2014, Masters et al., 2016, Chanda et al., 2017, Ortblad, Musoke et al., 2017, Gichangi et al., 2018), conducted between 2011 and 2018 and including 20,758 participants, met the eligibility criteria for inclusion in the review (Figure 3.1: Study flow diagram).

Figure 3.1. Flow Diagram through different phases of the review

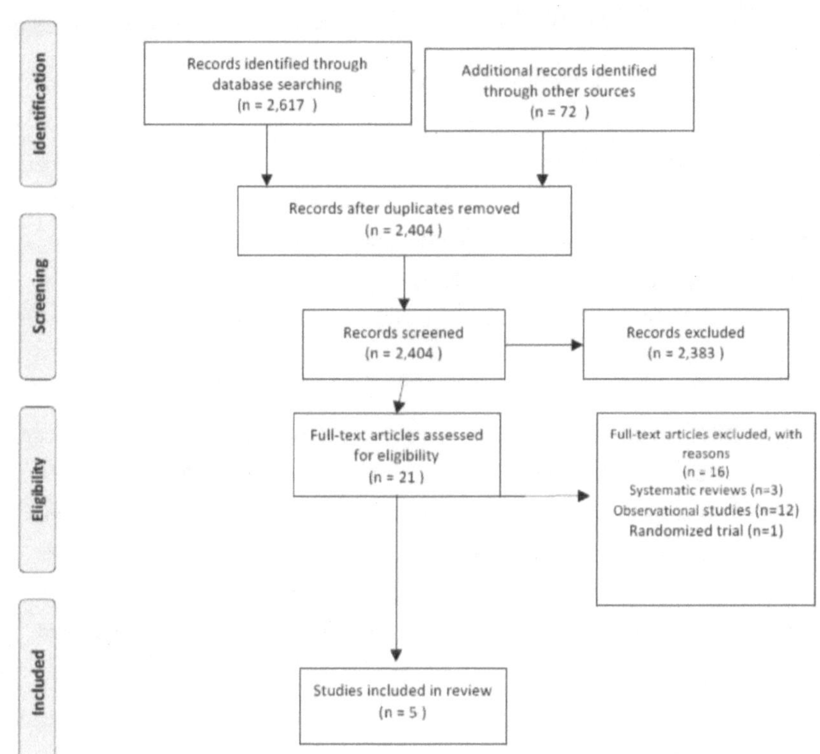

Figure 3.1. Study flow diagram

Five of the RCTs were reported in full-text articles (MacPherson et al., 2014, Masters et al., 2016, Chanda et al., 2017, Ortblad et al., 2017, Gichangi et al., 2018). Of the five RCTs, two were from Kenya (Masters et al., 2016, Gichangi et al., 2018), one from Zambia (Chanda et al., 2017), one from Uganda (Ortblad et al., 2017) and one from Malawi (MacPherson et al., 2014).

Four RCTs were primarily in urban settings (MacPherson et al., 2014, Masters et al., 2016, Chanda et al., 2017, Ortblad et al., 2017) and one study did not specify whether the study setting was urban or rural (Gichangi et al., 2016, Gichangi et al., 2018).

Two RCTs aimed to increase the uptake of HIV testing among male partners of pregnant women attending antenatal clinics or women attending postnatal clinics after the birth of a child (Gichangi et al., 2016, Masters et al., 2016, Gichangi et al., 2018). Another two RCTs were among female sex workers (Chanda et al., 2017). One RCT was conducted among adults aged 16 years and older from the general population (MacPherson et al., 2014, Chanda et al., 2017, Ortblad et al., 2017). Across all five RCTs, none reported on the yield of new HIV-positive diagnoses (one of our primary outcomes) and instead reported HIV positivity.

Four of the RCTs compared HIVST to standard HTS (Gichangi et al., 2016, Masters et al., 2016, Chanda et al., 2017, Ortblad et al., 2017, Gichangi et al., 2018). One RCT compared optional home-based confirmatory testing and initiation of antiretroviral therapy (ART) to HIVST accompanied with referral to facility-based HIV care services (MacPherson et al., 2014). All five RCTs used free oral fluid-based HIVST, followed by confirmatory HIV rapid diagnostic tests and none used finger stick/ or whole blood-based RDTs or both oral and blood specimens.

3.10.2 Excluded studies

There were 16 excluded studies, 12 of which were excluded based on their study design (i.e. observational studies), three systematic reviews and one trial, which did not report the outcomes of this review.

3.11 HIVST intervention compared with standard HIV testing services

3.11.1 Uptake of HIV testing

Two RCTs in Kenya (n=2,168) (Masters et al., 2016, Gichangi et al., 2018), assessed the uptake of HIV testing.

The studies recruited women, with no risk of intimate partner violence and with male partners of unknown HIV status or known HIV-negative status, at antenatal and postnatal care. Pregnant women were invited to either distribute HIV self-tests to their male partners (intervention arm) or an invitation card and referral vouchers for free HIV testing here assumed to be standard HIV testing services (comparison arm).

Two RCTs conducted in Zambia and Uganda (n= 1,925), recruited adult female sex workers, who reported the exchange of any vaginal, anal, or oral sex for money, goods, or other items of value (Chanda et al., 2017, Ortblad et al., 2017). The participants were invited to either direct delivery of HIVST or coupons free collection of HIVST (intervention arms) or referral for standard HIV testing services (control arm). Meta-analysis showed an increase in the uptake of HIV testing in the direct delivery of HIVST arm compared with the standard HTS arm (RR = 3.46, 95% CI: 1.62 to 7.37; $Tau^2 = 0.55$; $Chi^2 = 328.54$; df= 3($p < 0.00001$; $I^2 = 99$ %) The I^2 of 99 % is the proportion of the variation in observed effects due to variation of the true effects (Figure 3.2).

Study or Subgroup	HIVST Events	HIVST Total	Standard of care Events	Standard of care Total	Weight	Risk Ratio M-H, Random, 95% CI
Chanda et al.,2017a	265	295	226	301	26.8%	1.20 [1.11, 1.29]
Masters et al.,2016	258	297	148	303	26.7%	1.78 [1.57, 2.01]
Gichangi et al.,2018	322	472	132	471	26.6%	2.43 [2.08, 2.85]
Ortbland et al., 2017a	279	297	5	303	19.9%	56.93 [23.86, 135.85]
Total (95% CI)		**1361**		**1378**	**100.0%**	**3.46 [1.62, 7.37]**
Total events	1124		511			

Heterogeneity: $Tau^2 = 0.55$; $Chi^2 = 328.54$, df = 3 ($P < 0.00001$); $I^2 = 99\%$

Test for overall effect: Z = 3.21 (P = 0.001)

Risk Ratio M-H, Random, 95% CI: 0.1 0.2 0.5 1 2 5 10 — Standard of care HIVST

Figure 3.2. Forest plot: HIVST versus standard HIV testing services among male partners of pregnant women and female sex workers; outcome: Uptake of HIV testing.

Meta-analysis including two RCTs among pregnant women showed an increase in the uptake of couples HIV testing in the HIVST arm compared to standard HTS, (RR = 2.64, 95% CI: 2.01 to 3.47; $Tau^2 = 0.03$; $Chi^2 = 4.62$; df= 1(P=0.03; $I^2 = 78\%$). Couples HIV testing referred to the participant and her male partner testing together at the same time. The I^2 of 78% is the proportion of the variation in observed effects due to variation of the true effects (Figure 3.3).

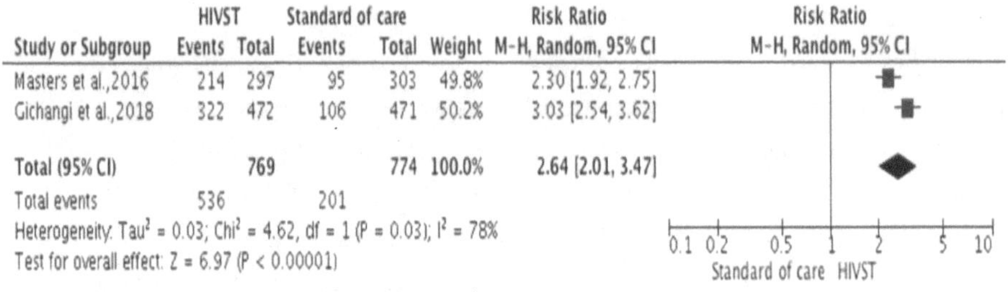

Study or Subgroup	HIVST Events	HIVST Total	Standard of care Events	Standard of care Total	Weight	Risk Ratio M-H, Random, 95% CI
Masters et al.,2016	214	297	95	303	49.8%	2.30 [1.92, 2.75]
Gichangi et al.,2018	322	472	106	471	50.2%	3.03 [2.54, 3.62]
Total (95% CI)		**769**		**774**	**100.0%**	**2.64 [2.01, 3.47]**
Total events	536		201			

Heterogeneity: $Tau^2 = 0.03$; $Chi^2 = 4.62$, df = 1 (P = 0.03); $I^2 = 78\%$
Test for overall effect: Z = 6.97 (P < 0.00001)

Risk Ratio M-H, Random, 95% CI
0.1 0.2 0.5 1 2 5 10
Standard of care HIVST

Figure 3.3. Forest plot: HIVST versus standard HIV testing services among male partners of pregnant women; outcome: Uptake of couples HIV testing.

3.11.2 HIV positivity

Three RCTs assessed HIV positivity among male partners of pregnant women (two studies) and female sex workers following HIV testing (one study). HIV positivity rate was determined as a proportion of male partners or female sex workers diagnosed HIV-positive over those who accepted HIV testing. Meta-analysis showed no statistically significant difference in reporting HIV positivity among male partners of pregnant women and female sex workers from direct delivery of HIVST compared to standard HTS (RR = 0.94, 95% CI: 0.76to 1.16; $Tau^2 = 0.00$; $Chi^2 = 1.69$; df= 2(p < 0.43; $I^2 = 0$ %) The I^2 of 0 % is the proportion of the variation in observed effects due to variation of the true effects. Figure 3.4).

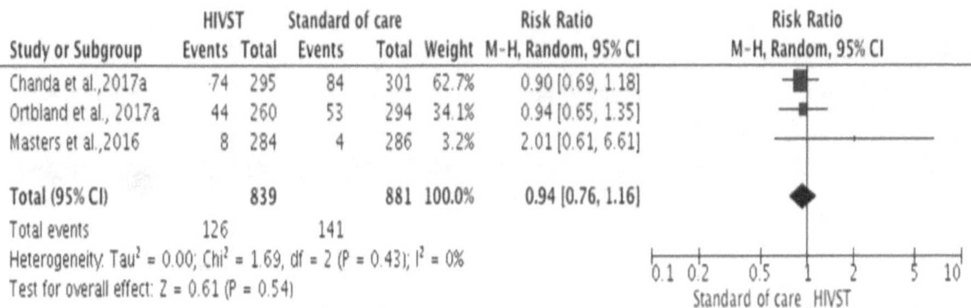

Study or Subgroup	HIVST Events	HIVST Total	Standard of care Events	Standard of care Total	Weight	Risk Ratio M-H, Random, 95% CI
Chanda et al.,2017a	74	295	84	301	62.7%	0.90 [0.69, 1.18]
Ortbland et al., 2017a	44	260	53	294	34.1%	0.94 [0.65, 1.35]
Masters et al.,2016	8	284	4	286	3.2%	2.01 [0.61, 6.61]
Total (95% CI)		**839**		**881**	**100.0%**	**0.94 [0.76, 1.16]**
Total events	126		141			

Heterogeneity: Tau^2 = 0.00; Chi^2 = 1.69, df = 2 (P = 0.43); I^2 = 0%
Test for overall effect: Z = 0.61 (P = 0.54)

Figure 3.4. Forest plot: HIVST versus standard HIV testing services among male partners of pregnant women and female sex workers; outcome: HIV positivity.

3.11.3 Linkage to ART

Three RCTs reported on linkage to ART care among HIV positive male partners of pregnant women (one study) and female sex workers (two studies). Meta-analysis showed that participants from direct delivery of HIVST are less likely to seek HIV–related care and initiating ART compared to participants from HTS (RR = 0.72, 95% CI: 0.57 to 0.91; Tau^2 = 0.00; Chi^2 = 1.34; df= 2(p < 0.51; I^2 = 0 %) The I^2 of 0 % is the proportion of the variation in observed effects due to variation of the true effects. Figure 3.5.

Study or Subgroup	HIVST Events	HIVST Total	Standard of care Events	Standard of care Total	Weight	Risk Ratio M-H, Random, 95% CI
Masters et al.,2016	2	8	3	4	3.1%	0.33 [0.09, 1.26]
Chanda et al.,2017a	35	74	54	84	66.4%	0.74 [0.55, 0.98]
Ortbland et al., 2017a	27	80	24	53	30.4%	0.75 [0.49, 1.14]
Total (95% CI)		**162**		**141**	**100.0%**	**0.72 [0.57, 0.91]**
Total events	64		81			

Heterogeneity: Tau^2 = 0.00; Chi^2 = 1.34, df = 2 (P = 0.51); I^2 = 0%
Test for overall effect: Z = 2.73 (P = 0.006)

Risk Ratio
M-H, Random, 95% CI
0.1 0.2 0.5 1 2 5 10
Standard of care HIVST

Figure 3.5. Forest plot: HIVST versus standard HIV testing services among male partners of pregnant women and female sex workers; outcome: Linkage to ART treatment.

3.11.4 Social harms

Three RCTs assessed any type of social harms following HIVST or standard HTS among HIV positive male partners of pregnant women (one study) and female sex workers (two studies). Masters et al. (2016) in Kenya reported a single incident of harm in each group between two HIV-negative participants in the HIVST group and the control group. In both groups, the reported harm was verbal and/ or physical IPV (Masters et al., 2016). Chanda et al. (2017) in Zambia reported four incidences of harm, with three participants in the direct delivery of HIVST intervention arm and one participant in the coupons intervention arm, reporting physical violence following primary partner learning of their HIVST use. No incident of harm was reported in the standard of care arm (Chanda et al., 2017). Ortblad et al.(2017) in Uganda reported four incidents of harm, with one participant in the direct delivery of HIVST intervention arm and one participant in the coupons intervention arm, reporting verbal abuse following primary partner learning of their HIVST use/or mental distress following a positive HIVST result. Two participants in the standard of care arm reported verbal abuse after disclosure of their HIV status

3.12 HIVST with optional home-initiation of HIV care compared to HIVST with facility-based HIV care

One RCT in Malawi (n=16,660) compared different approaches to HIVST (MacPherson et al., 2014). Before the HIVST intervention, counsellors promoted the availability of HIVST by door-to-door campaigning and distribution of leaflets in all 14 clusters. Participants in the intervention group who requested HIVST received free oral Quick rapid test kits from the house of trained volunteer counsellors to perform HIVST with an optional home-initiation of HIV care, after pre-test counselling, instructions and demonstration. Participants were offered the opportunity to test in the privacy of their own home and asked to return the used kits in person to the counsellor in a sealed envelope. Participants in the control group received self-test kits supplemented by facility-based HIV care at a clinic. All participants reported a positive HIV self-test result could go by themselves or be referred by the counsellors to study clinics.

In the arm with the offer of home ART initiation, study nurses conducted home visits for participants reporting a positive HIV self-test result and requesting optional home initiation of care following appointment organized by counsellors. Nurses performed confirmatory HIV testing, WHO staging, CD4 cell count, TB screening and 2 weeks ART to eligible participants. In the facility group, study nurses provided standard HIV care, including confirmatory HIV testing, WHO staging, CD4 cell count, TB screening and onward referral for ART initiation to participants with a positive HIV self-test result attending any of the three study clinics (Table 3.1).

3.12.1 HIV positivity

The trial reported HIV positivity among participants following HIV testing. HIV positivity was determined as the proportion of participants diagnosed HIV-positive over those who accepted HIV testing. The results showed that 6% (n=490/8194) of participants in the arm with the offer of optional home-based confirmatory testing and initiation of ART group reported a positive HIVST test result compared to 3.3% (n=278/8466) of participants in the facility group (RR: 1.86; 95% CI: 1.16 to 2.98; P= .010).

3.12.2 Testing for CD4 counts

MacPherson et al. (2014) also compared the receipt of CD4 count test results among newly diagnosed HIV-positive individuals. In the arm that offers optional home-based confirmatory testing and initiation of ART group, 72. 5 % (n=79/109) of newly diagnosed HIV positive individuals received CD4 count results compared to 51 % (n=23/63) in the facility group (RR= 0.70, 95% CI: 0.54 to 0.91; P= .007).

3.12.3 Linkage to ART treatment

MacPherson et al. (2014) also reported ART initiation and retention in care. In the arm with the offer of optional home-based confirmatory testing and initiation of ART group, initiation of ART was 37% (n=181/490) compared to 22.7 % (n=63/278) in the control arm (RR, 2.94; 95% CI: 2.10 to 4.12; P < .0001). After adjusting for reported household mortality at baseline, the effect of availability of home ART care was (ARR, 2.44; 95% CI: 1.61 to 3.68; P < .001).

Of the 181 ART initiators in the home group, 64% (n=116/181) initiated at home and 36% (n=65/181) initiated at 1 of the 3 health facilities. After 6 months, 28.7% (n=52/181) of ART initiators in the home group and 23.8% (n=15/63) of ART initiators in the facility group were lost from ART care. Participants in the home group were more likely to initiate ART but also more likely to be lost to ART at 6-month follow-up.

3.13 Assessment of risk of bias in included studies

The assessments of risk of bias in included studies are presented in the risk of bias graph below (Figure 3.6), while additional details are included in tables 3.1, 3. 2 and 3.3.

Because of the nature of the interventions, all included trials (n=5) were judged to be at high risk of performance bias and detection bias. This is because of unclear reporting on blinding of participants, personnel or outcome assessment (MacPherson et al., 2014, Gichangi et al., 2016, Masters et al., 2016, Chanda et al., 2017, Ortblad et al., 2017, Gichangi et al., 2018). One trial was judged to be at uncertain risk of reporting bias because the study did not report results of those in the intervention group, who did receive confirmatory HIV testing, and sexual behaviour and decision-making outcomes (Gichangi et al., 2016, Gichangi et al., 2018). One trial was judged to be at an uncertain risk of reporting bias because the study protocol was unavailable for a full review (Gichangi et al., 2018).

All included trials had a low risk of attrition bias because participant withdrawal rates were < 20 % (MacPherson et al., 2014, Gichangi et al., 2016, Masters et al., 2016, Chanda et al., 2017, Ortblad et al., 2017, Gichangi et al., 2018).

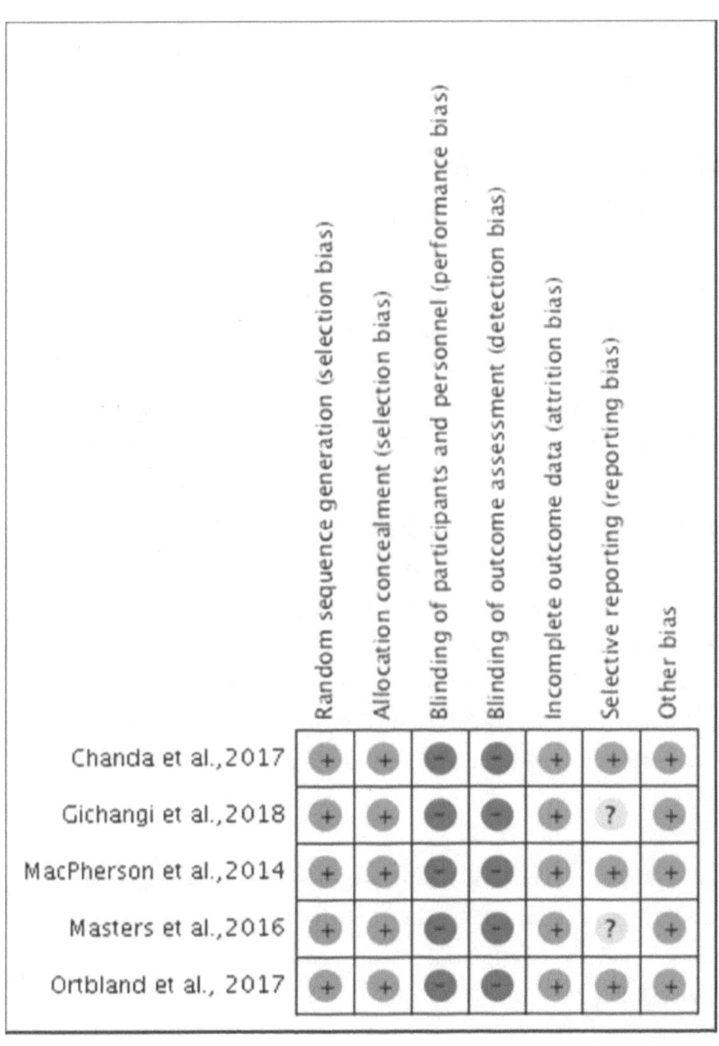

Figure 3.6. Risk of bias summary: review authors' judgments about each risk of bias item for each included study.

3.14 Assessment of overall quality of the evidence

We used the Grading of Recommendations Assessment, Development and Evaluation (GRADE) approach to assess the quality of evidence and generate absolute estimates of effect for the outcomes as described in the GRADE profiler (GRADEpro) software (Guyatt et al., 2008, Balshem et al., 2011). The GRADE methodology defines the quality of evidence for each outcome as 'the extent to which one can be confident that an estimate of effect or association is close to the quantity of specific interest." (Higgins and Green 2005). The quality rating across studies has four levels: high, moderate, low or very low. RCTs are initially categorized as providing high-quality evidence with the option of downgrading the quality. Quality of evidence can be downgraded based on limitations in design, indirectness of evidence, unexplained heterogeneity or inconsistency of results, imprecision of results or high probability of publication bias (Higgins and Green 2005). Downgrading was not done based on a lack of blinding alone because of difficulties of blinding participants and or research personnel in HIV testing intervention trials. We did not downgrade based on the risk of bias when lack of blinding was accompanied by additional high risks of bias (e.g., selection bias and incomplete outcome reporting). The quality of evidence for the studies separately for each outcome in the GRADE Summary of Findings is summarized below (Guyatt et al., 2008).

3.15 Overall quality of evidence

The overall quality of evidence for the four RCTs (Masters et al., 2016, Gichangi et al., 2018, Chanda et al., 2017, Ortblad et al.,2017), was moderate. The quality of evidence was downgraded because of the risk of performance bias, reporting bias, imprecision and inconsistency, as shown in Table 3.2.

able 3.2. HIV self-testing compared to the standard of HIV testing services for adults

atient or population: Pregnant women and post-natal women aged 18 years and above and their male partners.
ettings: Ante-natal clinics in urban settings in Africa
ntervention: HIV self-testing
omparison: Standard of HIV testing services

utcomes	**Illustrative comparative risks* (95% CI)**		**Relative effect (95% CI)**	**No of Participants (studies)**	**Quality of the evidence (GRADE)**
	Assumed risk	Corresponding risk			
	Standard of care	**HIV self-testing**			
ptake of HIV testing (direct delivery of HIVST versus standard of care)					
	371 per 1000	**1000 per 1000** (601 to 1000)	**RR 3.46** (1.62 to 7.37)	2739 (4 studies)	IJIJIJĴ **moderate**
ptake of HIV testing (coupon for free HIVST versus standard of care)					
	160 per 1000	**200 per 1000** (126 to 317)	**RR 1.25** (0.79 to 1.98)	2708 (4 studies)	IJIJIJĴ **moderate**
ptake of couple HIV testing					
	260 per 1000	**473 per 1000** (410 to 545)	**RR 1.82** (1.58 to 2.1)	1543 (2 studies)	IJIJIJĴ **moderate**
IV positivity (direct delivery of HIVST versus standard of care)					
	160 per 1000	**150 per 1000** (122 to 186)	**RR 0.94** (0.76 to 1.16)	1720 (3 studies)	IJIJĴĴ **low**
IV positivity (coupon for free HIVST versus standard of care)					
	160 per 1000	**200 per 1000** (126 to 317)	**RR 1.25** (0.79 to 1.98)	1756 (3 studies)	IJIJĴĴ **low**
tarted ART (direct delivery of HIVST versus standard of care)					
	574 per 1000	**414 per 1000** (322 to 513)	**RR 0.72** (0.57 to 0.91)	303 (3 studies)	IJIJĴĴ **low**
tarted ART (coupon for free HIVST versus standard of care)					
	574 per 1000	**506 per 1000** (396 to 643)	**RR 0.88** (0.69 to 1.12)	270 (3 studies)	IJIJĴĴ **low**

The basis for the **assumed risk** (e.g. the median control group risk across studies) is provided in footnotes. The **orresponding risk** (and its 95% confidence interval) is based on the assumed risk in the comparison group and the **elative effect** of the intervention (and its 95% CI).
I: Confidence interval; **RR:** Risk ratio;

RADE Working Group grades of evidence
igh quality: Further research is very unlikely to change our confidence in the estimate of effect.
oderate quality: Further research is likely to have an important impact on our confidence in the estimate of effect and ay change the estimate.
ow quality: Further research is very likely to have an important impact on our confidence in the estimate of effect and is kely to change the estimate.
ery low quality: We are very uncertain about the estimate.

Risk of bias: Downgraded the quality of evidence by 1 level for risk of bias. The outcome of HIV testing in all 4 trials as based on self-reporting and the risk of detection bias and performance bias cannot be excluded.
Inconsistency: Downgrading for inconsistency was not done, despite a high statistical heterogeneity. However, the stimates of effects were beneficial across all trials.
Indirectness: Did not downgrade for indirectness but note that two trails were conducted as couples testing of pregnant omen and their male partners and two other trails with female sex workers and their partners.
Imprecision: Did not for imprecision, despite a few numbers of events and a wide confidence interval around the estimate f the effect in one trial.
Risk of bias: Downgraded the quality of evidence by 1 level for risk of bias. The outcome of HIV testing in 2 trials was

based on self-reporting and the risk of detection bias and performance bias cannot be excluded.
[6] Inconsistency: Downgrading for inconsistency was not done, despite a high statistical heterogeneity. However, the estimates of effects were beneficial across the two trials.
[7] Risk of bias: Downgraded the quality of evidence by 1 level because the outcomes were self-reports and performance could not be excluded.
[8] Imprecision: Downgraded the quality of evidence by 1 level because of the event rate in both groups and a wide confidence interval around the estimate of effect.

The overall quality of the evidence for the cluster RCT (MacPherson, Lalloo et al. 2014) was moderate. The quality of evidence was downgraded because of the risk of performance and detection biases. Table 3.3.

Table 3.3. HIV self-testing with optional home initiation of HIV care compared to HIVST with facility-based HIV care services for adults					
Patient or population: Adults aged 16 years and above recruited from the general population. **Settings:** Urban settings in Africa **Intervention:** HIVST with optional home-based HIV care services **Comparison:** HIVST with facility-based HIV care services					
Outcomes	**Illustrative comparative risks* (95% CI)**		**Relative effect (95% CI)**	**No of Participants (studies)**	**Quality of the evidence (GRADE)**
	Assumed risk	Corresponding risk			
	Standard of care	**HIV self-testing**			
HIV positivity					
	524 per 1000	**524 per 1000** (440 to 623)	**RR 1.86** (1.16 to 2.98)	16660 (1 study)	IJIJIJʃ [1,2,3,4] **moderate**
Tested for CD4 count					
	33 per 1000	**54 per 1000** (23 to 124)	**RR 0.70** (0.54 to 0.91)	16660 (1 study)	IJIJIJʃ [1,2,3,4] **moderate**
Started ART					
	7 per 1000	**5 per 1000** (3 to 10)	**RR 1.86** (2.10 to 4.12)	16660 (1 study)	IJIJIJʃ [1,2,3,4] **moderate**
*The basis for the **assumed risk** (e.g. the median control group risk across studies) is provided in footnotes. The **corresponding risk** (and its 95% confidence interval) is based on the assumed risk in the comparison group and the **relative effect** of the intervention (and its 95% CI). **CI:** Confidence interval; **RR:** Risk ratio; **HR:** Hazard ratio;					
GRADE Working Group grades of evidence **High quality:** Further research is very unlikely to change our confidence in the estimate of effect. **Moderate quality:** Further research is likely to have an important impact on our confidence in the estimate of effect and may change the estimate. **Low quality:** Further research is very likely to have an important impact on our confidence in the estimate of effect and is likely to change the estimate. **Very low quality:** We are very uncertain about the estimate.					
[1] Risk of Bias: Downgraded one level for performance and detection bias as neither providers nor participants, or outcome assessors were blinded (Macpherson et al., 2105). [2] Inconsistency: Cannot be appraised in a single study. [3] Indirectness: We did not downgrade of indirectness but note that the findings are from one trial. [4] Imprecision: No serious imprecision was noted.					

3.16 Discussion

3.16.1 Summary of main results

The objective of this systematic review was to synthesize the evidence on the effects of HIVST among adults in Africa on the uptake of testing, the yield of new HIV–positive diagnoses, linkage to ARV treatment and the incidence of social harms. This review included five RCTs with male partners of pregnant and post-partum women and adults in the general population in Malawi, Kenya, Zambia and Uganda.

Two models of HIV testing were assessed in the included studies of this review. The first model included four RCTs comparing HIVST versus standard HTS and the second model included one RCT comparing different approaches to HIVST. In the first model, four RCTs in Kenya, Zambia and Uganda found a positive effect on the uptake of HIVST compared to standard HTS. Similarly, the two RCTs in Kenya reported a positive effect on the uptake of couples' HIVST compared to standard HTS.

Three RCTs in Kenya, Zambia and Uganda reported no statistically significant difference in reporting HIV positivity among male partners of pregnant women and female sex workers from HIVST compared to standard HTS. Conversely, the same three RCT reported an increase in linkage to ART care among HIV positive male partners of pregnant women and female sex workers from standard HTS compared with those from HIVST. Finally, seven (7) incidences of any kind IPV were reported following HIVST and standard HTS from four RCTs in Kenya, Zambia and Uganda.

In the second model, one RCT in Malawi reported a statistically significant difference; showing participants who received HIVST and an optional home-based confirmatory testing and initiation of ART were more likely to report HIV positive test results than those in the control group. Further, the RCT showed an increased proportion of newly diagnosed HIV positive participants in the home group received CD 4 count test than those in the control group.

Finally, the trial reported a statistically significant difference showing that participants who reported HIV-positive test results from home-based HIVST with optional home-based confirmatory testing and initiation of ART were more likely to initiate ART care compared with their counterparts from the home-based HIVST with facility-based HIV care.

3.17 Summary of evidence: HIVST versus standard of HIV testing services

3.17.1 Uptake of HIVST

Four RCTs were included in the meta-analysis and showed the moderate quality of evidence for the uptake of HIV testing compared to standard HTS. Furthermore, two RCTs were included in the meta-analysis also showed the moderate quality of evidence for uptake of couple HIV testing. Although the results of the meta-analysis report that HIVST can double the uptake of HIV testing compared to standard HTS, there is some uncertainty because of heterogeneity in effect size between the studies. Also, the evidence was limited to male partners of pregnant and post-partum women and adult female sex workers.

3.17.2 HIV positivity

Three RCTs included in this review with moderate evidence showed no difference between HIVST compared to standard HTS in reporting HIV-positivity. The quality of evidence was downgraded for risk of bias, detection bias, selection bias and imprecision. None of the RCTs reported a yield of new HIV-positive diagnoses. Yield and HIV positivity are important for designing appropriate and sustainable HIV testing interventions because they determine the number of tests needed to diagnose a new case of HIV and has cost and resource implications (Govindasamy et al., 2015). However, none of the RCTs included in this review reported on the yield of new HIV positive diagnoses, underscoring the need to assess this important indicator in future studies, particularly in high HIV prevalence settings.

3.17. 3 Linkage to HIV care

Three trials from Kenya, Zambia and Uganda, included in this review with moderate evidence showed poor linkage to HIV care following confirmatory testing between HIV positive participants in the HIVST group compared to those in the standard HTS group (Masters et al., 2016, Chanda et al., 2017, Ortblad et al., 2017).

3.17.4 Social harms

One RCT from Kenya, compared distribution of HIVST kits by pregnant women to their male partners with standard HTS and 2 RCTs from Zambia and Uganda compared delivery of HIVST kits with standard HTS among adult female sex workers and assessed IPV resulting from HIVST. The RCTs reported seven incidences of any form of IPV reported by pregnant women and female sex workers, related to HIV self-testing (Masters et al., 2016, Chanda et al., 2017, Ortblad et al., 2017). Self-testing may alter IPV experiences, but the extant literature currently does not accurately measure it. This finding of reported rare cases of IPV related to HIVST is consistent with several studies assessing harm across all forms of HTS (WHO 2012, Brown et al., 2014, Choko et al., 2015). However, it is important to introduce HIVST with caution among vulnerable populations e.g. female sex workers [FSW] (Thirumurthy et al., 2016, WHO 2016).

3.18 Summary of evidence: comparison of different approaches to HIVST

3.18.1 HIV positivity

One RCT from Malawi with moderate-quality evidence, assessed different approaches to HIVST and observed that participants from home-based HIVST with optional home-based confirmatory testing and initiation of ART were significantly more likely to report a positive result than participants from home-based HIVST with facility-based HIV care (MacPherson et al., 2014).

3.18.2 Tested for CD 4 count

The same RCT in Malawi, with moderate-quality evidence, showed a high proportion of newly diagnosed HIV-positive participants from home-based HIVST optional home-based confirmatory testing and initiation of ART compared to participants from home-based HIVST with facility-based HIV care who had tested for CD4 counts (MacPherson et al., 2014).

3.18.3 Started ART

Additionally, the same RCT in Malawi with moderate evidence reported a higher ART initiation in those with home-based HIVST with optional home-based confirmatory testing compared with their counterparts from the home-based HIVST with facility-based HIV care. However, this RCT reported a loss to follow-up 6 months after home-initiation of ART compared with facility-initiation of ART. ART initiators in the home group had higher rates of loss from ART compared with their counterparts in the facility group.

3.19 Overall completeness of the evidence and applicability of evidence

The observed results on increased uptake concur with results from other systematic reviews (Krause et al., 2013, Pai et al., 2013, Suthar et al., 2013, Figueroa et al., 2015, Johnson et al., 2017). For instance, the systematic reviews reported uptake of HIVST ranging from 50% to 96% in other parts of the world (Krause et al., 2013, Pai et al., 2013, Suthar et al., 2013) and 20% to 74 % in the key populations (Suthar et al., 2013, Figueroa et al., 2015).

Besides, observational studies from Kenya (Mugo et al., 2017) Lesotho, (Zerbe et al., 2015), Malawi (Choko et al., 2011, Choko et al., 2015) and Zimbabwe (Sibanda et al., 2016), reported similar increases in the uptake of HIV testing through HIVST.

For example, a two-year prospective study in Malawi reported a consistently high community-based HIVST uptake among adolescents aged 16-19 years of age; young people aged 16-29 years of age, women and men (Choko et al., 2015).

The RCTs also reported an increased uptake of couple's testing from HIVST compared with the approach of giving male partners invitation letters or vouchers for free HTS. These results suggest that men may be more likely to prefer HIVST than standard HTS (Harichund and Moshabela 2017).

This observation underscores the importance of getting men to utilize HTS because it is well documented that men compared with women are known to underutilize HTS and present late for care ending up with worse outcomes on treatment (Mukolo et al., 2013, The IeDEA and ART cohort collaborations 2014).

Observational studies among key populations, including men who have sex with men [MSM] (Figueroa et al., 2015), people who inject drugs [PWIDs] or people who use drugs [PWUDs] (Sharma et al., 2015) and female sex workers (Cowan 2016) , revealed high HIV testing uptake following the offer of HIVST. Existing evidence suggests that to achieve universal knowledge of HIV status, it is imperative to have innovative interventions such as HIVST to increase access to HIV testing. This review confirms that HIVST is an important strategy to improve awareness of HIV status among adults in Africa, particularly SSA and provides an additional HIV testing option to conventional approaches such as VCT, PITC, school-based and workplace testing to reach untested populations (Sharma et al., 2015, WHO 2016).

Earlier HIV diagnosis supports timely access to ART, with several beneficial consequences, such as improved life expectancy, reduced HIV transmission, decreased stigma related to HIV testing and provision of HIV prevention interventions (Johnson et al., 2017).

These results are consistent with results from observational studies among the general populations in SSA, which reported HIV-positivity ranging from 3 to 14% (Choko et al., 2015, Mavedzenge et al., 2016, Sibanda et al., 2016, Thirumurthy et al., 2016) and from 1 to 30 % among key populations (Cowan 2016, Thirumurthy et al., 2016). As coverage of HIV testing increases, the proportion of HIV-positive test and new HIV-positive diagnoses will be likely to decrease and hence calls for more focused HIV testing methods to continue to achieve the same or higher levels of HIV-positivity (Sharma et al., 2015, WHO 2016). This review identified gaps in the evidence on linkage to care. Linkages to further HIV testing and HIV prevention, treatment and care services are a critical component in the HIV testing cascade.

This is more important in HIVST because it requires linkage to confirmatory testing, particularly among those who report a positive HIV test result (Johnson et al., 2017). The most probable explanation for the observed low level of linkage could be due to a few diagnosed HIV-positives, under-reporting and the possibility that some men were aware of their HIV-positive status and already in care. Innovative follow-up strategies post HIVST such as use of mobile phones or short message services, or facilitated HIV care assessments and ART initiation interventions could encourage linkage (Choko et al., 2015, Sharma et al., 2015, WHO 2016, Johnson et al., 2017).

HIV testing experts recognize the importance and complexity of monitoring, reporting, evaluating and mitigating social harms related to HIV testing. The rare cases of social harm related to HIVST reported in this review, help to alleviate a major concern of HTS experts, regarding IPV related to HIVST.
The finding may suggest that HIVST does not directly influence the risk of IPV, but the risks are largely context-specific, including the settings (e.g. urban/rural) and relationship dynamics of couples and partners.

To emphasize this critical concern, the WHO recommends that HIV testing programmes consider context-specific strategies to implement HIV testing approaches, including HIVST (WHO 2016, Harichund and Moshabela 2017).

Furthermore, fear of status disclosure or stigma, the possibility of false-positive diagnoses, lack of confirmatory HIV testing and insufficient quality control procedures highlight the need to address legal and human rights issues related to HIVST (WHO 2012, WHO 2016, Johnson et al., 2017).

3.20 Quality of the evidence

According to the GRADE system, well-conducted RCTs provide high-quality evidence, while observational studies provide low-quality evidence. This review included only RCT data and we found the quality of evidence reported from 4 RCTs for the HIVST versus standard HTS was generally moderate. The model for comparison of different approaches for HIVST, including one high-quality RCT provided moderate quality of evidence.

3.21 Potential biases in the review process

We used a broad search strategy to capture as many studies as possible. We limited our search to those studies conducted in Africa from 1998 to date to improve comparability. A random-effects model was used to pool data. Despite using a broad search strategy, we were able to capture five RCTs conducted across four countries in SSA. The limited number of RCTs that were included in this review may have affected the overall sample size and affected the confidence in the pooled estimates. Further, there are limited studies from other parts of Africa, which may limit the generalizability of the review findings.

Additionally, we could not explain the 'heterogeneity' of effects, because we did not undertake sensitivity and sub-group analysis to determine the prediction interval and present the range of effects due to a small number (n=5) of RCTs included in this review. The review, therefore, cannot exclude the possibility that of the dispersion presented, what proportion is due to variance in true effects rather than sampling error (Borenstein et al., 2017). Publication bias was not formally assessed because of the limited number of RCTs, since analytical methods such as funnel plots and funnel plots asymmetry tests were not appropriate (Higgins and Green 2005).

3.22 Agreements and disagreements with other studies or reviews

To the authors' knowledge, this is the first systematic review evaluating the effects of HIVST on the uptake of HIV testing, linkage to ARV treatment and social harms among adults in Africa. Previous reviews focused on HIVST strategies, acceptability of HIVST and different community-based HIV testing approaches globally. The findings of this review provide important information on the potential of HIVST as an option for HTS among adults in Africa. A key finding of our review is that the uptake of HIVST is promising among male partners of pregnant women and adults in the general populations in Africa, particularly in SSA. Most important is the observation of high participation by male partners in couples' HIV testing through HIVST. However, more data is needed on a yield of new HIV-positive diagnoses, particularly from countries with high HIV prevalence in SSA in terms of the diverse range of context and settings.

Further research among key populations such as MSM, PWIDs/PWUDs, FSWs and vulnerable populations such as adolescents and men who have never tested for HIV and factors associated with their participation or non-participation in HIVST, is important to inform policy and practice. Further key areas for research include the effectiveness of HIVST in detecting previously undiagnosed HIV infection, or the number of repeat non-testers, linkage to care following a reactive self-test result or a confirmatory positive test, retention of care among those identified HIV-positive.

Other research areas are linkage to prevention services among participants with negative results (e.g. male circumcision) and social harms from HIVST, which are important to help guide policy on HIVST in Africa. Interventions to facilitate timely linkage to care post HIVST are ongoing in Zimbabwe (PACTR20160700171788) and Malawi (ISRCTN18421340), with preliminary findings reporting significant benefits on linkage to VMMC and ART using financial and non-financial incentives.

3.23 Implication for research

This review has reported moderate-quality evidence for the uptake of HIVST, suggesting that self-testing is an innovative strategy having the potential to increase uptake of HIV testing and increase awareness of HIV status among undiagnosed adults in Africa, particularly in SSA. We also reported no statistically significant difference in reporting HIV positivity between participants from HIVST and conventional HTS, indicating a need for further research particularly in high HIV prevalence settings in Africa. This review recommends that high-quality evidence from trials would provide valuable insight on whether HIVST is an additional HIV testing option. HIVST could facilitate early detection, early linkage to HIV care, treatment and prevention. Additional trial findings will provide data on HIVST as an invaluable tool for health authorities of African governments to increase access to HIV care, treatment and prevention to achieve the "95-95-95" global target by the year 2030 (UNAIDS 2018).

ole 3.1. Study and intervention characteristics of five RCTs (n=5).Ā

First author	Study design /Sample characteristics	Comparison condition	Intervention condition	Findings	Quality of evidence
isters, Agot et al. 2016)	Two - arm randomized controlled trial (1:1). 758 pregnant and post-partum women aged between 18 and 39 years in urban & peri-urban, Kenya, presenting at post-partum or antenatal care, with no risk of IPV and who had a male partner with unknown HIV status or known HIV-negative status.	Facility-based HIV testing (n= 303 male partners): Participants received an invitation card plus a voucher inviting their male partners for free HIV testing at study clinic. Women participants also received information on clinical counselling and legal support on IPV. The invitation cards had messages about the importance of testing.	Unsupervised HIVST (n= 297 male partners): Participants received two free Oral Quick RDT with manufacturer's instructions to distribute to their male partner or to test as a couple, a demonstration on how to use the kits, clinical counselling on how to encourage their male partners to test and legal support on IPV.	**Primary outcome:** **Uptake of HIV testing [a]:** Participants reported at follow-up the uptake of HIV testing by their male partner 36 weeks after her enrollment.86.7% Intervention Group (IG) vs. 52 % Control Group (CG) [Risk ratio (RR) =1.78; 95% Confidence Interval (CI): 1.57 to 2.01]. **Uptake of couples HIV testing [b]:** Participants reported uptake of couples HIV testing 36 weeks after enrolment. Couples testing referred to testing together at the same time.72.1 % IG vs. 31.3 % CG [RR=2.30; 95% CI: 1.92 to 2.75]. **HIV positivity [c]:** Participants self-reported that their male partners tested HIV-positive. 3.1 % IG vs. 2.7 % CG [RR=2.01; 95% CI: 0.61 to 6.61].	**Sequence generation:** Participants were randomized in a 1:1 ratio using computer-generated random numbers and using balanced block randomization (block size of 20) to HIVST group or a comparison. **Allocation concealment:** Participants were offered sealed randomized envelopes sequentially. **Blinding of participants and personnel:** The study did not describe the blinding process. After randomization, it was not possible to blind given the nature of the intervention and the comparison groups. **Blinding of outcome**

				<u>Secondary outcome:</u> **Social harm** [d]: Participants reported whether they experienced physical, emotional, verbal, or sexual violence from their partner after enrolment. 0.34 % (n=1/297) IG vs. 0.33% (n=1/303) CG	The study primarily relied on self-reported of outcomes from women of male partners who self-tested. The tracking number of referral vouchers at study facilities validated confirmatory testing following HIVST reactive results. **<u>Incomplete outcome data:</u>** The attrition rate was 5 % (Follow-up was completed for 95% of study participants (n=570/600). **<u>Selective reporting:</u>** Reported nearly all outcomes except confirmatory HIV testing results and sexual behaviour and decision-making outcomes. **<u>Other potential sources of bias:</u>** None
First author	**Study design /Sample characteristics**	**Comparison condition**	**Intervention condition**	**Findings**	**Quality of evidence**
ıangi et al. 3	Three-arm randomized controlled trial (1:1:1), however this review only includes the	Facility- based HIV testing (n= 471 male	Unsupervised HIVST (n= 472 male partners).	**<u>Primary outcome:</u>** **Uptake of HIV testing**	**<u>Sequence generation:</u>**

	comparison between two of the arms. The third arm was excluded from this review; it involved PMTC services. 1,410 pregnant women aged 18 years and older attending their first antenatal clinic visit, not at risk of IPV and 1,333 male partners with unknown or known HIV-negative status in Eastern & Central Kenya. Only 943 were included in the two arms under review.	partners): Women participants received a standard invitation letter to their male partner for HIV testing alone/ or as a couple at a standard of HIV testing care at the clinic.	Women participants' received an improved invitation letter emphasizing the importance of male HIV testing and 2 free Oral Quick RDT with manufacturer's instructions, to distribute to their male partner to test for HIV alone/or to test as a couple. <u>Women</u> participants also viewed 10 min. demonstration on how to use the kits and interpret the results correctly and were counselled on how to encourage their male partners to test and handle their male partners in case of a positive result.	[a]: Women participants reported uptake of HIV testing at 12 weeks follow-up by reporting if their male partner had an HIV test since she was enrolled in the study. 78.8 % IG vs. 28.2 % CG (# 2) [RR= 2.23; 95% CI: 2.08 to 2.85]. **Uptake of couples HIV testing [b]:** Women participants reported uptake of couples HIV testing at follow-up by reporting that they had tested together with her partner at the same time. 68. 4 % IG vs. 22.3 % CG (#2) [RR= 3.03 95% CI: 2.54 to 3.62].	Participants were randomly assigned using three different colours: Arm 1 was yellow, arm 2 was green and the arm was blue. Coloured stickers were labelled following each facility's sample size and put in sealed envelopes and mixed up. **<u>Allocation concealment:</u>** After consenting participants were asked to pick a sealed envelope and open. Participants were allocated to respective arms determined by the label colour they have picked. **<u>Blinding of participants and personnel:</u>** Study staffs were not blinded to knowing the study group to which each participant was randomized. Participants knew what they are being offered without

t author	Study design /Sample characteristics	Comparison condition	Intervention condition	Findings	Quality of evidenceĀ
					study staff. **Blinding of outcome assessment:** Self-reporting of outcomes by female participants and male participants who tested for HIV in all study arms. **Incomplete outcome data:** The study reported high retention rate for women participants (arm 1= 86%, arm 2=83%, arm 3 = 84%). Male partner follow-up was also high (arm 1=80%, arm 2 =76%, arm 3=84%). Intent-to-treat analysis was done at 3-months. **Selective reporting:** The study protocol was unavailable for a full review. **Other potential sources of bias:** None noted

nda et al., 7	Three-arm randomized controlled trial (1:1:1), Peer educators enrolled 965 female sex workers aged 18 years of age or older in 3 Zambian transit towns.	Facility-based HIV testing (n= 320 female sex workers): Participants received information about existing HIV testing services from peer-educators, including the locations and working hours, where they could obtain an HIV test.	1. Direct delivery of HIVST kit (n= 316 female sex workers): Participants received 2 Oral Quick RDT HIVST kits. Peer educators distributed 2 HIVST kits during their intervention visits to participants in the community (one at the 1st visit (week 0); a second one at the fourth visit (10th week), with manufacturer's pictorial and written instructions in English and 3 local languages. Peer-educators demonstrated to participants on how to use the kit, results interpretation and follow-up care. 2. Distribution of a coupon (n= 329 female sex workers). Participants received a coupon from trained peer-educators for a free Oral Quick RDT HIVST kit from a health facility or pharmacy. Peer-educators distributed the 2 coupons at the 1st and 4th intervention	**<u>Primary outcome:</u>** **Uptake of HIV testing** [a]**:** Participants self-reported uptake of HIV testing at 1 month and 4-month study assessments **<u>At 1 month:</u>** 94.9 % IG (1) vs. 88.5 % CG [RR= 1.07; 95% CI: 0.99 to 1.15]; 84.4 % IG (2) vs. 88.5 % CG [RR= 0.95; 95% CI: 0.86 to 1.05]. **<u>‡At 4 months:</u>** 84.1 % IG (1) vs. 75. 1 % CG [RR=1.20; 95% CI: 1.11 to 1.29]; 79.8 % IG (2) vs. 75. 1% % CG [RR=1.25; 95% CI: 1.16 to 1.34]. **HIV positivity** [c] **:** Participants self-reported that their most recent HIV test was positive. **<u>At 1 month:</u>** 16.7 % IG (1) vs. 20. 5 % CG [RR= 0.78; 95% CI: 0.51 to 1.02]; 12.4 % IG (2) vs. 20.5 % CG [RR= 0.75; 95%	**<u>Sequence generation:</u>** The randomization list was computer generated in random blocks of size 3, 6 and 9 and stratified by 3 study sites to ensure balance in study arms by the site. **<u>Allocation concealment:</u>** Participants were sequentially allocated into one of the three study arms using sealed opaque, sequentially numbered envelopes. **<u>Blinding of participants and personnel:</u>** Due to the nature of the intervention, masking was not possible; however, the peer educator's study arm assignment was concealed until all participants had been enrolled.

			community. The content of the test and instructions were identical to those in the delivery arm.	**♯At 4 months:** 25.3 IG(1) vs. 28.2 % CG [RR= 0.91; 95% CI: 0.70 to 1.19]; 25.7 % IG (2) vs. 28.2 % CG [RR= 0.90; 95% CI: 0.69 to 1.18]. **Started ART[e]:** Participants with an HIV –positive test result self-reported that they were taking antiretroviral medicines. **At 1 month:** 22. 5% IG(1) vs. 46.6 % CG [RR= 0.55 ; 95% CI: 0.27 to 1.10]; 25 % IG (2) vs. 46.6 % CG [RR= 0.62; 95% CI: 0.30 to 1.30]. **♯At 4 months:** 48 % IG (1) vs. 64.3% CG [RR= 0.74; 95% CI: 0.55 to 0.98]; 57.1% IG (2) vs. 64.3 % CG [RR= 0.89; 95% CI: 0.66 to 1.14]. **Secondary outcome:** **Social harm[i]** Physical, sexual, or verbal intimate partner	**Blinding of outcome assessment:** Due to the nature of the intervention, the masking was not done. **Incomplete outcome data:** Attrition rate : at 1 month= 9%; at 4 months= 7 % **Selective reporting:** Reported results of all (1= primary; 4= secondary) study outcomes **Other potential sources of bias:** None detected.

				violence, unintentional disclosure of HIV status, or self-harm (self-reported). 0.6% (n= 2/316) IG (1) vs. 0.6 % (n= 2/329) IG (2). No adverse events were reported in the standard of care arm	
t author	**Study design /Sample characteristics**	**Comparison condition**	**Intervention condition**	**Findings**	**Quality of evidence**
›lad et al., 7.	Three-arm randomized controlled trial (1:1:1), Peer educators enrolled 960 female sex workers aged 18 years of age or older in 5 Kampala divisions, Uganda.	Facility-based HIV testing (n= 328 female sex workers): Participants received information about existing HIV testing services, including the locations and working hours, from peer-educators.	1. Direct delivery of HIVST (n= 296 female sex workers): Peer educators distributed 2 HIVST kits during their intervention visits to participants in the community (social networks) one at the 1st visit (week 0); a second one at the fourth visit (10th week), with manufacturer's pictorial and written instructions in English and Luganda - a local language. Peer-educators demonstrated to participants on how to use the kit, interpretation of results and follow-up care. Participants also received free condoms. 2. Distribution of a coupon (n= 336 female	**Uptake of HIV testing [a]:** Participants self-reported uptake of HIV testing at 1 month and 4 month study assessments **<u>At 1 month:</u>** 95.2 % IG (1) vs. 71.5 % CG [RR= 1.33; 95% CI:1.17 to 1.51]; 80.4 % IG (2) vs. 71.5 % CG [RR= 1.12; 95% CI: 0.96 to 1.32] **<u>♯At 4 months:</u>** 99.6 % IG (1) vs. 87.1 % CG [RR= 56.93; 95% CI: 23.86 to 135.85]; 97 % IG (2) vs. 87.1 % CG [RR= 59.67; 95% CI: 25.02 to 142.35]. **HIV positivity [c] :** Participants self-reported that their most recent HIV test was positive.	**<u>Sequence generation:</u>** The randomization list was computer generated in random blocks of size 3, 6 and 9 and stratified by 5 administrative divisions and evenly recruited peers to ensure balance in study arms by the site. **<u>Allocation concealment:</u>** Participants were sequentially allocated into one of the three study arms using opaque, sequentially numbered envelopes. **<u>Blinding of participants and</u>**

			sex workers). Participants received a coupon from the trained peer-educators to collect a free 2 Oral Quick RDT HIVST kit from 10 private health facility or pharmacy in exchange for the coupon. Peer-educators distributed the 2 coupons at the 1st and 4th to the participants during the intervention visits in the community (social networks). The content of the test and instructions were identical to those in the delivery arm.	**<u>At 1 month:</u>** 13.6 % IG (1) vs. 13 % CG [RR= 1.05; 95% CI: 0.62 to 1.75]; 17.3 % IG (2) vs. 13 % CG [RR= 1.27; 95% CI: 0.74 to 2.19]. **<u>♯At 4 months:</u>** 16.9 % IG (1) vs. 18 % CG [RR= 0.94; 95% CI: 0.65 to 1.35]; 27.7 % IG (2) vs. 18 % CG [RR= 1.54; 95% CI: 1.13 to 2.09]. **Started ART[e]:** Participants with an HIV –positive test result self-reported that they were taking antiretroviral medicines. **<u>At 1 month:</u>** 4.5 % IG (1) vs. 4.3 % CG [RR= 0.99; 95% CI: 0.37 to 2.67]; 3.2 % IG (2) vs. 4.3 % CG [RR= 0.76; 95% CI: 0.29 to 2.02]. **<u>♯At 4 months:</u>** 7.3 % IG (1) vs. 8.2 % CG [RR= 0.75; 95% CI: 0.49 to 1.14]; 9.3 % IG (2) vs. 8.2 % CG [RR= 0.95; 95%	**<u>personnel:</u>** Due to the nature of the intervention, masking was not possible; however study personnel, peer educators and participants were masked to study arm assignment before opening the sealed envelopes. **<u>Blinding of outcome assessment:</u>** Due to the nature of the intervention, the masking was not done. **<u>Incomplete outcome data:</u>** The study reported high retention rate for women participants. Attrition rate was: at 1 month= 4 %; at 4 months= 8.5 % **<u>Selective reporting:</u>** Reported results of all (1 = primary; 6=secondary) study outcomes. **<u>Other potential</u>**

				CI: 0.61 to 1.52]. **Secondary outcome:** **Social harm**[d]**:** Participants were screened for physical, sexual, or verbal intimate partner violence, unintentional disclosure of HIV status and self-harm at each peer educator intervention visit and during study assessments. 0.7 % (n= 2/296) IG (1) vs. 0.6 % (n= 2/336) IG (2). No adverse events were reported in the standard of care arm	**sources of bias:** None detected
t author	**Study design /Sample characteristics**	**Comparison condition**	**Intervention condition**	**Findings**	**Quality of evidence**
Pherson et 014	Two-arm cluster randomized controlled trial (1:1) 16,660 adults aged 16 years and above recruited from 14 clusters in urban Blantyre Malawi. All 14 clusters were restricted randomized into 2 groups: HIVST with optional home initiation of HIV care services or HIVST with facility-based HIV care services only.	Unsupervised home-based HIV ST with facility-based standard HIV care services (n= 8,466): Adult participants' who requested HIVST received free Oral Quick test kits. Participants who reported HIV positive results could self-refer or referred by the counsellor to study clinics for confirmatory HIV	Unsupervised home-based HIVST with optional home initiation of HIV care services (n=8,194): Adult participants' who requested HIVST received free Oral Quick RDT from the house of volunteer counsellors to perform HIVST and pre-testing information, counselling and demonstration on how to use the kits.	**Secondary outcomes:** **HIV positivity** [c]**:** Participants self-reported that their most recent HIV test was positive. 6 % IG vs. 3.3 % CG [RR= 1.86, 95 % CI: 1.16 to 2.98]. **Linkage to care** [f]**:** Participants with an HIV –positive test result self-reported that they have sought medical care for their	**Sequence generation:** Reported that 14 clusters were randomized in a 1:1 ratio (7 clusters into intervention group; 7 clusters into the control group). **Allocation concealment:** Used coloured balls from an opaque bag held above eye level to select the

		ART at 1 of the 3 study facilities. ART initiation was ascertained by interviewing all adults who initiated ART at any of the 3 study clinics.	the used kit in person to the counsellor in a sealed envelope after self-testing. Participants had an option to report or not to report their self-test results to the counsellor. Counsellors organized home visits by study nurses for participants reporting a positive HIV self-test result who requested home initiation of HIV care. ART initiation was ascertained by recording all adults who initiated ART at home.	(i)**CD 4 counts** [g]**:** 72.5 % IG vs. 51 % CG [RR= 0.70, 95 % CI: 0.54 to 0.91]. (ii)**Started ART**[e]**:** Participants with an HIV –positive test result self-reported that they were taking antiretroviral medicines. 2.2 % IG vs. 0.7 % CG [RR=2.94, 95% CI: 2.10 to 4.12]*.	clusters and allocation. **Blinding of participants and personnel:** Reported blinding of investigators but not the counsellors, or study participants, or outcome assessors. **Blinding of outcome assessment:** Due to the nature of the study masking was not done. **Incomplete outcome data:** All participants completed the trial, the attrition rate was 28.7 % in IG and 23.8 % in CG from ART, no treatment withdrawals, no trial group changes and no major adverse events reported. **Selective reporting:** The study reported results of all outcomes (1 primary; 4 secondaries).

					Other potential sources of bias: None detected.

intervention group; CG= control group; IPV=intimate partner violence; PMCT= Prevention-of-mother-to-child-transmission; [a] Proportion of participants offered HIV testing underwent HIV testing; [b] Proportion of participants who undergo HIV testing with their partners; [c] Proportion of participants with a reactive self-test that received irmatory testing and diagnosed HIV positive over those who accepted HIV testing; [d] Proportion of self-reported instances of intimate partner violence, self-harm, or coercion st for HIV; [e] Proportion of participants who have received confirmatory testing and diagnosed HIV positive self-reporting taking ART medicines over those with an HIV-tive results

portion of participants with an HIV-positive test result self-reporting whether they had sought medical care for their HIV infection;

sed on WHO criteria (CD4 $\leq$ 350 cells μl); [h] Proportion of all resident adults who initiate ART during the first 6 months of the home-based HIV-testing intervention. *The minator is all study participants, not HIV positive participants; ♯ data used in meta-analysis.Ā

References

Balshem, H., M. Helfand, H. J. Schunemann, A. D. Oxman, R. Kunz, J. Brozek, et al. (2011). "GRADE guidelines: 3. Rating the quality of evidence." Journal of Clinical Epidemiology **64**(4): 401-406.

Borenstein, M., J. P. Higgins, L. V. Hedges and H. R. Rothstein (2017). "Basics of meta-analysis: I2 is not an absolute measure of heterogeneity." Research Synthesis Methods **8**(1): 5-18.

Brown, A. N., E. W. Djimeu and D. B. Cameron (2014). "A Review of the Evidence of Harm from Self-Tests." AIDS Behavior **18: S445–S449**.

Chanda, M. M., K. F. Ortblad, M. Mwale, S. Chongo, C. Kanchele, N. Kamungoma, et al. (2017). "HIV self-testing among female sex workers in Zambia: A cluster randomized controlled trial." PLoS Medicine **14**(11): e1002442.

Choko, A. T., N. Desmond, E. L. Webb, K. Chavula, S. Napierala-Mavedzenge, C. A. Gaydos, et al. (2011). "The Uptake and Accuracy of Oral Kits for HIV Self-Testing in High HIV Prevalence Setting: A Cross-Sectional Feasibility Study in Blantyre, Malawi." PLoS Medicine **8**(10).

Choko, A. T., P. MacPherson, E. L. Webb, B. A. Willey, H. Feasy, R. Sambakunsi, et al. (2015). "Uptake, Accuracy, Safety and Linkage into Care over Two Years of Promoting Annual Self-Testing for HIV in Blantyre, Malawi: A Community-Based Prospective Study." PLoS Medicine **12**(9): e1001873.

Choko, A. T., P. MacPherson, E. L. Webb, B. A. Willey, H. Feasy, R. Sambakunsi, et al. (2015). "Uptake, Accuracy, Safety and Linkage into Care over Two Years of Promoting Annual Self-Testing for HIV in Blantyre, Malawi: A Community-Based Prospective Study." PloS Medicine **12**(9): e1001873.

Cowan, F. (2016). Designing safe, acceptable and appropriate HIVST interventions for female sex workers. 21st International AIDS Conference, Durban, South Africa.

Eisinga, A., N. Siegfried and M. e. a. Clarke (2007). "The sensitivity and precision of search terms in Phases I, II and III of the Cochrane Highly Sensitive Search Strategy for identifying reports of randomized trials in Medline in a specific area of health care-HIV/AIDS prevention and treatment interventions." Health Information and Library Journal **24**: 103-109.

Figueroa, C., C. Johnson, A. Verster and R. Baggaley (2015). "Attitudes and Acceptability on HIV Self-testing Among Key Populations: A Literature Review." AIDS and Behavior: 1-17.

Fylkenes, K. and S. Siziya (2004). "A randomized trial on the acceptability of voluntary counselling and testing." Trop Med Int Health **9**(5): 566-572.

Gichangi, A., J. Wambua, S. Mutwiwa, R. Njogu, E. Bazant, J. Wamicwe, et al. (2018). "Impact of HIV Self-Test Distribution to Male Partners of ANC Clients: Results of a Randomized Controlled

Govindasamy, D., R. A. Ferrand, S. M. Wilmore, N. Ford, S. Ahmed, H. Afnan-Holmes, et al. (2015). "Uptake and yield of HIV testing and counselling among children and adolescents in sub-Saharan Africa: a systematic review." Journal of International AIDS Society **18**: 20182.

Govindasamy, D., K. Kranzer, N. van Schaik, F. Noubary, R. Wood, R. P. Walensky, et al. (2013). "Linkage to HIV, TB and non-communicable disease care from a mobile testing unit in Cape Town, South Africa." PLoS ONE **8**(11): e80017.

Guyatt, G. H., A. D. Oxman, V. G.E., R. Kunz, Y. Falck-Ytter and P. Alonso-Coello, et al. (2008). "GRADE: an emerging consensus on rating quality of evidence and strength of recommendations." BMJ **336**: 924-926.

Harichund, C. and M. Moshabela (2017). "Acceptability of HIV Self-Testing in Sub-Saharan Africa: Scoping Study." AIDS Behavior **22**: 560-568.

Higgins, J. P. T. and S. Green (2005). Cochrane handbook for Systematic Reviews of Interventions 4.2.5 (updated May 2005).

Johnson, C., R. Baggaley, S. Forsythe, H. van Rooyen, N. Ford, S. Napierala Mavedzenge, et al. (2014). "Realizing the Potential for HIV Self-Testing." AIDS Behav Doi 10.1007/s10461-014-0832-x.

Johnson, C., R. Baggaley, S. Forsythe, H. van Rooyen, N. Ford, S. Napierala Mavedzenge, et al. (2014). "Realizing the Potential for HIV Self-Testing." AIDS Behavior.

Johnson, C. C., C. Kennedy, V. A. Fonner, N. Siegfried, C. Figueroa, S. Dalal, et al. (2017). "Examining the effects of HIV self-testing compared to standard HIV testing services: a systematic review and meta-analysis." Journal of the International Aids Society **20**(1).

Krause, J., F. Subklew-Sehume, C. Kenyon and R. Colebunders (2013). "Acceptability of HIV self-testing: a systematic literature review." BMC Public Health **13:**(735.): 1-19.

Lee, V. J., S. C. Tan, A. Earnest, P. S. Seong, H. H. Tan and Y. S. Leo (2007). "User acceptability and feasibility of self-testing with HIV rapid tests." Journal of Acquired Immune Deficiency Syndromes **45**(4): 449-453.

MacPherson, P., D. G. Lalloo, E. L. Webb, H. Maheswaran, A. T. Choko, S. D. Makombe, et al. (2014). "Effect of Optional Home Initiation of HIV Care Following HIV Self-testing on Antiretroviral Therapy Initiation Among Adults in Malawi: A Randomized Clinical Trial." Jama **312**(4): 372-37

Mahler, H. R., B. Kileo, K. Curran, M. Plotkin, T. Adamu, A. Hellar, et al. (2011). "Voluntary Medical Male Circumcision: Matching Demand and Supply with Quality and Efficiency in a High-Volume Campaign in Iringa Region, Tanzania." PLoS Medicine **8**(11): 1-8.

Masters, S. H., K. Agot, B. Obonyo, S. Napierala Mavedzenge, S. Maman and H. Thirumurthy (2016). "Promoting Partner Testing and Couples Testing through Secondary Distribution of HIV Self-Tests: A Randomized Clinical Trial." PLoS Medicine **13**(11): e1002166.

Mavedzenge, S. N., E. Sibanda, Y. Mavengere, J. Dirawo, K. Hatzold, O. Mugurungi, et al. (2016). Acceptability, feasibility and preference for HIV self-testing in Zimbabwe. 21st International AIDS Conference, Durban, South Africa, July 18-22, 2016.

Mugo, P. M., M. Micheni, J. Shangala, M. H. Hussein, S. M. Graham, T. F. Rinke de Wit, et al. (2017). "Uptake and Acceptability of Oral HIV Self-Testing among Community Pharmacy Clients in Kenya: A Feasibility Study." PLoS ONE **12**(1): e0170868.

Mukolo A., Villegas R., Aliyu M. and W. K. A. (2013). "Predictors of late presentation for HIV diagnosis: a literature review and suggested way forward." AIDS and Behavior **17(1)**: 5-30.

NASCOP (2008). Guidelines for HIV Testing and Counselling in Kenya. Nairobi, Kenya, National AIDS and STI Control Programme Ministry of Public Health and Sanitation, Kenya.

Njau, B., M. Werfalli, L. Abdullahi and C. Mathews (2016). "A systematic review on uptake and yield of HIV self-testing among adults in Africa." Retrivied from ÂČČÆĖĎĎĎ ĖĆYĒĄĆĀĖĊĀĖMOLMCOLĠOC O KBCKEĖYÃÆĂVĖĊĄĆYĖĈÆĖĄAOBÎ ÌĤHĪ ĤÌÍÍÍ Ĩ.

Ortblad, K., D. K. Musoke, T. Ngabirano, A. Nakitende, J. Magoola, P. Kayiira, et al. (2017). "Direct provision versus facility collection of HIV self-tests among female sex workers in Uganda: A cluster-randomized controlled health systems trial." PLoS Medicine **14**(11): e1002458.

Pai, N. P., J. Sharma, S. Shivkumar, S. Pillay, C. Vadnais, L. Joseph, et al. (2013). "Supervised and Unsupervised Self-Testing for HIV in High- and Low-Risk Populations: A Systematic Review." PLoS Medicine **10(4):** : e1001414. .

Piennar, E., L. Grobler and K. Busgeeth, et al, (2011). "Developing a geographic search filter to identify randomized controlled trials in Africa: finding the optimal balance between sensitivity and precision." Health Information and Library Journal **28**: 210-215.

Review Manager [RevMan] (2014). The Nordic Cochrane centre, The Cochrane Collaboration. Review Manager(RevMan). Version 5.3 for Windows. Copenhagen: The Nordic Cochrane centre, The Cochrane Collaboration,2014.

SAHIVSOC (2012). "Joint statement on HIV testing and counselling." Retrieved 20/4/2015, from ÂČČÆĖĎĎĎ ĖVÂÃÇĈĄXĖĄĆÁĖÅZĎĈĄĄÅĖ society-news.

Sharma, M., et al., (2015). "Systematic review and meta-analysis of community and facility-based HIV testing to address linkage to care gaps in sub-Saharan Africa." Nature **528**: S77-S85.

Sharma, M., R. Ying, G. Tarr and R. Barnabas (2015). "Systematic review and meta-analysis of community and facility-based HIV testing to address linkage to care gaps in sub-Saharan Africa." Nature **528**(7580): S77-85.

Sibanda, E., M. Mutseta, K. Hatzold, S. Gudukeya, A. Dhliwayo, C. Lopez, et al. (2016). Community-based distribution of HIV self-test kits: results from a pilot of door-to-door distribution of

HIV self-test kits in one rural Zimbabwean community. 21st International AIDS Conference, Durban, South Africa.

STAR (2015). "HIV Self-Testing Africa Initiative-Research." from [illegible].

Suthar, A. B., N. Ford, P. J. Bachanas, V. J. Wong, J. S. Rajan, A. K. Saltzman, et al. (2013). "Towards Universal Voluntary HIV Testing and Counselling: A Systematic Review and Meta-Analysis of Community-Based Approaches." PLoS Medicine **10(8):**(e1001496.).

The IeDEA and ART cohort collaborations (2014). "Immunodeficiency at the start of combination antiretroviral therapy in low-, middle- and high-income countries." Journal of Acquired Immune Deficiency Syndromes **65(1): e8–e16**.

Thirumurthy, H., S. H. Masters, S. N. Mavedzenge, S. Maman, E. Omanga and K. Agot (2016). "Promoting male partner HIV testing and safer sexual decision making through secondary distribution of self-tests by HIV-negative female sex workers and women receiving antenatal and post-partum care in Kenya: a cohort study." Lancet HIV **3**: e266–274.

UNAIDS (2013). Global report: UNAIDS report on the global AIDS epidemic 2013.In.Geneva, Switzerland.

UNAIDS (2014). The GAP Report. Geneva, Switzerland.

UNAIDS (2014). UNAIDS Gap Report 2014, Geneva, Switzerland.

UNAIDS (2015). HOW AIDS CHANGED EVERYTHING: MDG 6: 15 YEARS, 15 LESSONS OF HOPE FROM THE AIDS RESPONSE, JOINT UNAIDS & WHO, Geneva Switzerland.

UNAIDS (2018). Global AIDS Update 2018: Miles To Go Closing Gaps Breaking Barriers Righting Injustices.

UNAIDS/WHO (2004). UNAIDS/WHO Policy Statement on HIV Testing., Geneva: United Nations Programme on HIV/AIDS(UNAIDS)and World Health Organization(WHO).

Walensky, R. P. and I. V. Bassett (2011). "HIV Self-testing and the Missing Linkage." PLoS Medicine **8**(10): 1-2.

Walensky, R. P., E. Losina, K. A. Steger-Craven and K. A. Freedberg (2002). "Identifying Undiagnosed Human Immunodeficiency Virus: The Yield of Routine, Voluntary Inpatient Testing." Archive of Internal Medicine **162(8)** 887-892.

Walensky, R. P., R. Wood, M. O. Fofana, N. A. Martison and L. E. e. al. (2010). "The Clinical Impact and Cost-effectiveness of Routine Voluntary HIV screening in South Africa." Journal of Acquired Immune Deficiency Syndromes.

WHO (1998). Health expectancy is more important than life expectancy-Message from the WHO Director-General on the World Health Report 1998. Geneva, Switzerland, WHO.

WHO (2012). HIV service delivery approaches to HIV testing and counselling(HTC): a strategic HTC programme framework., World Health Organization.

Wong, V., C. Johnson, E. Cowan, M. Rosenthal, R. Peeling, M. Miralles, et al. (2014). "HIV Self-Testing in Resource-Limited Settings: Regulatory and Policy Considerations." AIDS Behavior **18 Suppl 4**: S415-421.
World Health Organization (2016). Guidelines on HIV self-testing and partner notification: supplement to consolidated guidelines on HIV testing services. France., World Health Organization, Geneva 27, Switzerland.: 1-104.
Zerbe, A., A. L. DiCarlo, J. E. Mantell, R. H. Remien, D. D. Morris, K. Frederix, et al. (2015). Acceptability and Uptake of Home-Based HIV Self-Testing in Lesotho. 19th Conference on Retroviruses and Opportunistic Infections, Seattle, Washington, USA.

CHAPTER FOUR

4.0 Qualitative evidence synthesis

4.1 A systematic review of qualitative evidence on factors enabling and deterring uptake of HIV self-testing in Africa

4.2 Introduction

HIV is a serious public health burden in Africa, particularly in sub-Saharan Africa (SSA). More than 75% of HIV infected people are in Africa and nearly half (45.7%) of newly diagnosed cases of HIV among adults are among Africans. Efforts to achieve the global target of 95-95-95 by 2030 requires increased uptake of HIV testing as an entry point to the HIV cascade (UNAIDS 2017, UNAIDS 2018, UNAIDS 2019). HIV Self-Testing (HIVST) has been introduced as an innovative tool with the potential for reaching high-risk populations, including young people and enabling them to know their sero status and facilitate linkage to care for those who test HIV positive (Johnson et al., 2017).

Globally, systematic reviews on HIVST provided evidence on motivators for, barriers to and preferences to HIVST (Krause et al., 2013, Pai, Sharma et al., 2013, Suthar et al., 2013, Johnson et al., 2017). Key motivators reported include convenience, short testing and waiting time, privacy, autonomy/sense of self-empowerment and, perceived control of one's health choices. Besides, the reviews reported a high preference for rapid oral fluid tests compared to blood-based testing, indicating preference for a simple, less invasive procedure, compared with needle sticks used to draw blood samples (Krause et al., 2013, Pai et al., 2013, Suthar et al., 2013, Johnson et al., 2017). Other advantages of oral fluid HIV tests are easy to sample collection and acquisition, a minimum waiting time of 20 minutes before getting a result and reduction of needle stick injuries.

Additional advantages are low viral load in oral fluids and safer waste materials disposal (Krause et al., 2013, Pai et al., 2013, Suthar et al., 2013, Johnson et al., 2017). Literature from studies conducted globally report various HIVST related barriers.

Most barriers are crosscutting including lack of policies on HIVST, misperception on quality of self-test kits and perceived adverse effects associated with self-testing (Choko et al., 2011, Xun et al., 2013, Johnson et al., 2014, Njau et al., 2014).

The current evidence on facilitators of and barriers to HIVST uptake however, is from studies conducted in high-income settings, with few studies from Africa. Despite WHO recommendation for the introduction of HIVST as a strategy to increase universal coverage of HIV testing services (HTS), most African countries lag in terms of integration of HIVST in their national HTS policy. HIV policymakers have reservations about the introduction of HIVST and raise concerns ranging from lack of policies and regulatory systems, quality of HIVST kits, ethical and human rights issues and knowledge gaps about HIVST (Wong et al., 2014, Wong et al., 2019). To address these gaps, we conducted this study to review the existing qualitative evidence on the factors, which may enable or deter the uptake of HIVST among adults in Africa.

4.3 Objectives

The objectives of the systematic review of qualitative evidence were to identify, appraise and synthesize the evidence from qualitative studies on HIV stakeholders' and potential adult users' perceptions about factors that enable or deter the uptake of HIVST and to identify, appraise and synthesize adult users' experiences of HIVST in Africa.

4.4 Methods

This is a systematic review of qualitative evidence (i.e. qualitative evidence synthesis) and the unit of analysis will be the reviewed published articles article.

Two authors independently screened the search output, selection of the studies and data extraction. Any discrepancies were resolved by consensus and discussion. The authors used the Critical Appraisal Skills Programme (CASP) quality assessment tool for qualitative studies.

4.4.1 Search strategy

We searched for related studies in CINAHL, MEDLINE in Pubmed, EMBASE, AJOL, PsycINFO, Social Science Citation Index (SSCI) and Web of Science electronic databases using guidelines developed by the Cochrane Qualitative Research Methods Groups for searching for qualitative evidence (Noyes et al., 2009). Besides, we searched for related articles and grey literature, contacted experts in the field and scanned reference lists of studies related to barriers, facilitators and HIV self-testing experiences. For barriers and facilitators, we used search terms for Boolean search strategy such as " adult", "HIV", "Human Immunodeficiency Virus", "AIDS", "Acquired Immunodeficiency Syndrome", "self-testing", "HIV self-testing", "HIVST", "barriers", "facilitators", "HIV self-testing experiences, "Africa", "Africa South of the Sahara". A comprehensive search strategy for Medline was developed to ensure that all relevant literature was captured (Appendix C). Modification of the search strategy was done for other databases. All abstracts were saved using the Endnote reference manager software. We used various combinations of these terms with the search engines.

4.5 Inclusion and exclusion criteria

Studies were eligible if qualitative research methods (qualitative interview, focus group discussions and systematic observations) were used to explore factors that enable or deter the uptake of HIVST and testing experiences of adult users. The populations of interest were HIV stakeholders such as HIV policymakers, HIV experts, health care providers and adult users of HIVST.

Because of language constraints, studies not published in English were excluded. Conference abstracts were included only if they represented original qualitative data.

4.6 Data collection

4.6.1 Data extraction and management

A data extraction form designed specifically for this synthesis was used to extract data (Appendix D). The form was used to extract key themes and categories relevant to the synthesis objectives. The categories were derived during the initial phase of data extraction, including information on HIV stakeholders' perceptions of barriers to and facilitators for the uptake of HIVST and HIVST experiences of adult users. We extracted the researcher's interpretations, presented in the form of themes, concepts or categories from the results sections of the primary studies. We also perused the discussion sections and extracted as data relevant and well-supported researcher's interpretations. Additional information extracted included the first author's name, date of publication, language, country of study, context (urban, rural), participant group, the HIVST approaches studied, theoretical or conceptual frameworks applied and the study methodology. Two authors reviewed titles and abstracts in duplicate to exclude ineligible articles independently. Articles that met the inclusion criteria were selected for full-text review (Figure 4.1).

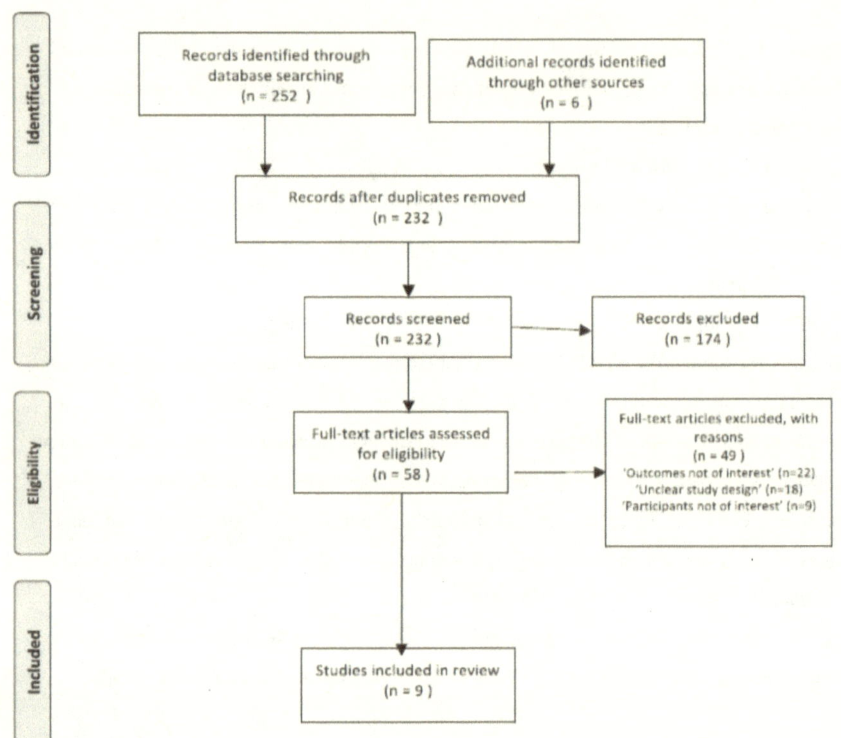

Figure 4.1. Flow diagram through different phases of the review

4.7 Quality assessment of included qualitative studies

The CASP -quality assessment tool- was used to assess the methodological quality (or limitations) of the qualitative studies (CASP 2014). Three primary studies were included in a pilot trial to assess the adequacy of the assessment tool and the integrity of the assessment.

One reviewer applied the appraisal framework to each included study. A second reviewer checked for discrepancies.

The assessment of methodological quality (or limitations) was not used to exclude studies but instead to determine the comparative contribution of each included study. The aim was to understand how each study contributed to the development of explanations and relationships and as part of the assessment of confidence in each review finding.

4.8 Assessment of confidence in the review findings

Each review finding from the included qualitative studies was assessed using the GRADE-Confidence in the Evidence from Reviews of Qualitative research (GRADE-*CERQual:* the certainty of qualitative evidence) approach (Lewin et al., 2018). *CERQual* was used to transparently access and describe how much confidence to place in the review findings. In the *CERQual* approach, four key components assess the certainty of qualitative evidence:

(a) The methodological quality of individual studies is the extent to which there are concerns about the design or conduct of the primary studies that contributed evidence to an individual review finding (Lewin et al., 2015, Lewin et al., 2018, Munthe-Kaas et al., 2018). The methodological limitations of the included studies contributing to each review finding were assessed using the modified CASP tool described above.
(b) The coherence of the review finding is an assessment of how clear and cogent (i.e. well supported or compelling) the fit is between the underlying data from the primary studies and a review finding that synthesizes that data (Lewin et al., 2015, Colvin et al., 2018, Lewin et al., 2018).

The coherence of each review finding was assessed by exploring to what extent clear patterns could be identified across the data contributed by each study. Further, we sought plausible explanations if variations across studies existed.

(c) Adequacy of the data is an overall determination of the degree of richness and quantity of data contributing/or supporting a review finding (Lewin et al., 2015, Glenton et al., 2018, Lewin et al., 2018). The adequacy of the data for each review finding was assessed in terms of the "thickness" of data, the number of studies and the stratification of countries and/or regions.

(d) The relevance of included studies to the review question is the extent to which the body of evidence from the primary studies supporting a review question applies to the context specified in the review question (Lewin et al., 2015, Lewin et al., 2018, Noyes et al., 2018). The relevance of each review finding to the research question was assessed in terms of perspective or population, a phenomenon of interest, settings, place, intervention and findings.

After assessing each of the four components, we reported as having: minor, moderate, serious methodological limitations; no or very minor, moderate, serious concerns about coherence; very thin or thin data, moderate rich adequacy of data and unclear, partial, direct relevance. For the overall confidence, we used four levels to indicate the confidence of the qualitative evidence: high, moderate, low and very low (Lewin et al., 2015, Lewin et al., 2018). Our judgments were based on an initial assumption that all review findings were 'high confidence' and then downgraded by one, two or three levels if there were important rather than minor concerns regarding any of the four CERQual components. The summary table provides key findings, the confidence of evidence for each finding and an explanation of the assessment of the certainty of the qualitative evidence (CASP 2014).

4.9 Analysis and synthesis process

Thematic synthesis for HIV self-testing experiences, enablers of and deterrents to the uptake of HIVST was conducted using framework analysis (Britten et al., 2002, Campbell et al., 2003, Thomas and Harden 2008, Barnett-Page and Thomas 2009, Merten et al., 2010). The thematic analysis suits studies with predefined aims and objectives specifically to inform policy and health-related practice. The thematic synthesis aimed to identify 'barriers' and 'facilitators' to the uptake of HIVST and heightened understanding of HIVST users' experiences. The framework analysis consisted of four analysis steps (a) Familiarization, (b) Thematic framework, (c) Indexing and (d) Charting (Thomas and Harden 2008, Barnett-Page and Thomas 2009).

Familiarization: Two reviewers independently read and re-read the selected qualitative studies and recorded initial impressions related to the aims and objectives of the review.

Thematic framework: Two reviewers independently identified key themes across studies by combining the results and interpretations from individual primary studies. Thereafter, the two reviewers developed a coding scheme after consultations.

Indexing: The two reviewers systematically applied codes to the textual data. They also checked for discrepancies in coding as the analysis progressed.

Charting: Data was rearranged according to the appropriate coding and themes were summarized in tabular format regarding the primary studies. This process helped reviewers to view the data by themes and sub-themes and explore if there were any differences or similarities in the barriers, facilitators and HIVST users' experiences identified (Thomas and Harden 2008, Barnett-Page and Thomas 2009).

The framework analysis steps with explanations are summarized in Table 4.1 below.

Table 4.1. Framework analysis steps and an explanation of each step	
Analysis step	Explanation
1. Familiarisation	Two reviewers independently read and re-read selected primary studies, recording initial impressions related to the aim and objectives of the review.
2. Thematic framework	Themes were identified and the two reviewers developed a coding scheme after consultations.
3. Indexing	The two reviewers applied codes to the whole data set systematically after checking for discrepancies in coding.
4. Charting	Data was rearranged by code and themes were summarized in a tabular format regarding the primary studies, enabling reviewers to view data by themes and sub-themes.
Source: Developed by the author	

This qualitative synthesis of evidence is reported following the ENTREQ statement guidelines to ensure transparency (Tong et al., 2012).

Ethical considerations

This study did not undertake any formal data collection involving any humans or animals.

4.10 Results

4.10.1 Database Search

Two hundred and fifty eight papers were found across the three databases and 232 articles remained after excluding duplicates. One hundred and seventy-four articles were excluded because they did not meet the inclusion and exclusion criteria. We retrieved full texts for the remaining 58 articles. Out of 58 full-text articles assessed for eligibility, 49 articles were excluded because of the following: 'outcome not of interest' (n= 22), 'unclear study design' (n= 18) and 'participant not of interest' (n= 9). Nine studies met the inclusion criteria and were included in this synthesis (see Figure 4.1).

4.10.2 Study characteristics

The nine studies involved 397 participants and were conducted in five (5) countries, namely in Malawi, South Africa, Tanzania, Kenya and Zimbabwe. The studies were conducted in 2011 (n=1), 2013 (n=3), 2015 (n= 2), 2016 (n= 2) and 2017(n=1). The studies used a mixed-sex sample (n= 6), female only sample (n= 2) and male-only sample (n= 1). Studies were conducted with actual HIVST users (adult men and women in the general population (n = 2), potential HIVST users (adult men and women in the general population (n = 3), HIV stakeholders (e.g. HIV experts, HIV policymakers, researchers, ethicists, etc.) and healthcare providers (n= 3) and pregnant women attending the antenatal clinic and their male partners (n= 1). All of the included studies were published in peer-reviewed journals. Overall, studies provided some description of the selection of participants and data collection techniques and data analysis, although the descriptions were brief (Table 4.2).

ɔle 4.2.Characteristics of included studies (n= 9).

thor (year of study)	Country	Study aim	Study design and Participants per methods	Summary of findings
ıu et al., (2014)	Tanzania	To identify characteristics of HIV testing options associated with individuals' preferences for HIV testing.	Study design: Qualitative design. Methods: In-depth interviews (IDIs): Men (n=3); Women (n = 5)* Focus group discussions (FGDs): Men (n=15); Women (n=17)* Analysis: A note based approach. * aged 18 years and older.	Self-test for HIV was perceived less feasible for scale-up due to the unfamiliarity of HIVST; lack of counselling and accuracy of test results were perceived barriers.
mwenda et al.,(2014)	Malawi	To explore factors shaping the decision-making of cohabiting couples who opted to self-test in Blantyre, Malawi.	Study design: Qualitative study. Methods: IDIs: Men (n=17) and Women (n=17)*. Analysis: Detailed content analysis. *aged 18 years and older	Gender roles and relationship dynamics may influence the implementation of community-based HIVST among couples.
:k et al .,(2014)	Kenya, Malawi, South Africa	To evaluate the usability of a wide variety of test features suitable for HIV self-test kits.	Study design: Mixed method approach design. Methods: IDIs: Women (n=150).* Analysis: A framework approach. *aged 18 years and older	Pictorial instructions, simple sample collection with integrated test components and easy steps for interpretation of results may facilitate the usability of HIVST.
.kusha et al., (2015)	South Africa	To explore attitudes, opinions and experiences among key stakeholders regarding HIVST in South Africa.	Study design: Qualitative study Methods: IDIs (n= 12)§ Analysis: Constant comparison method. §Key HIV stakeholders, including government officials, HIV experts and health care providers; gender distribution note reported.	HIVST has the potential to reach hard-to-reach groups, including men.
.nings et al., (2017)	Tanzania	To assess perceived cost advantages and disadvantages of using HIVST kits among infrequent and never HIV-	Study design: Mixed-method design. Methods: IDIs: Men (n= 23)*	Financial gains and losses influence men's decision process to HIVST; low fees or free HIVST, reduced travel time,

		Tanzania.	* aged 15 years and older.	lost from earning income may increase the uptake of HIVST.
ı Rooyen et al.,(2015)	Kenya, Malawi, South Africa	To assess the perceptions of HIVST among stakeholders in three sub-Saharan countries.	Study design: Qualitative study. Methods: IDIs: (n= 54). Analysis: Thematic analysis. §HIV policymakers, HIV experts and health care providers.	HIVST is an important complementary approach to existing conventional HIV testing services; contextual and operational evidence needed to contribute to normative WHO guidance.
ravudh et al., (2017)	Malawi & Zimbabwe	To identify young people's preferences for HIV-self-testing (HIVST) delivery, determine the relative strength of preferences and explore behaviours and perceptions underlying preferences.	Study design: Mixed-method design. Methods: IDIs: Men (n=7); Women (n= 8)* FGDs: Men (n=47); Women (n= 60)* Analysis: Framework analysis. *aged 16-25 years old.	Young people believe that home-based distribution of low price self-test kits may optimize HIVST services.
oko et al. (2017)	Malawi	To explore views regarding the acceptability of offering HIV-self test kits alone or in combination with linkage intervention to ANC attendees aimed at their male partners.	Study design: Qualitative study. Methods: IDIs: Men (n= 10) and Pregnant women (n= 10)* FGDs: Men (n= 18) and Pregnant women (n= 24)* Analysis: Simple descriptive content analysis. *aged 18 years and older.	Perceived highly acceptability of woman-delivered HIVST among pregnant women attending ANC and their male partners; HIVST was not likely to lead to adverse events (i.e., IPV); conditional financial incentives may motivate male partners to link into HIV care post-HIVST.
ight et al. (2017)	South Africa	To assess the perceived usability and acceptability of HIVST among lay users using several self-test prototypes.	Study design: Mixed-method study. Methods: IDIs: Men (n=23) and Women (n=27)* Analysis: Not reported. *lay users aged 18 years and older in rural and peri-urban settings.	Perceived highly acceptability and readiness in the context of prototypes influenced by usability and perceived needs. Perceived easiness-to-use, privacy, autonomy, ease access, widespread availability of

				test kits, low or free kits, emerged as important factors influencing acceptability and desirability.

4.10.3 Quality assessment of included qualitative studies

The quality assessment of included studies used standardized criteria based on the CASP tool, which examined 10 criteria. Study quality was scored according to the CASP critical score as follows: If the criterion was completely met, the study was awarded 2 points; if the criterion was partially met, the study was awarded 1 point; if the criterion was not applicable/unmet/not mentioned, the study was awarded 0 points. Finally, the study quality was classified accordingly. A total score of 20 were classed high quality, scores of 16 to 19 were classed as moderate quality and studies with scores ≤ 15 were classed as low quality.

None of the study findings were assessed to be of high quality because of a lack of information regarding the relationship between researchers and participants. All nine studies were categorized as moderate quality (total score =18-19), as shown in Table 4.3.

Table 4.3. CASP critical appraisal of studies included in this review (n= 9).

1st Author (year of study)	CASP criterion [1]									
	1	2	3	4	5	6	7	8	9	10	Total Score [2]
Njau et al., (2014)	2	2	2	2	2	1	2	1	2	2	18
Kumwenda et al.,(2014)	2	2	2	2	2	1	2	2	2	2	19
Peck et al .,(2014)	2	2	2	2	2	1	2	2	2	2	19
Makusha et al., (2015)	2	2	2	2	2	1	2	2	2	2	19
Jennings et al., (2017)	2	2	2	2	2	1	2	2	2	2	19
van Rooyen et al.,(2015)	2	2	2	2	2	1	2	2	2	2	19
Indravudh et al., (2017)	2	2	2	2	2	1	2	2	2	2	19
Choko et al., (2017)	2	2	2	2	2	1	2	2	2	2	19
Knight et al. (2017)	2	2	2	2	1	2	2	2	2	2	19

[1] CASP criterion: 1. Was there a clear statement of the aims of the research? 2. Is a qualitative methodology appropriate? 3. Was the research design appropriate to address the aims of the research? 4. Was the recruitment strategy appropriate to the aims of the

All of the included studies gave a clear statement of the aims of their research, using either in-depth interviews and/or focus group discussions. None of the studies used long-term ethnographic research.

Furthermore, none of the included studies discussed reflexivity (i.e. consideration of the relationship between the researchers, participants and study settings). Eight of the included studies had a description of data analysis and they used different analysis strategies, such as descriptive or exploratory approaches. Eight of the included studies had their findings supported by the data, except for one study with a relatively short description of the preference of HIVST among study participants. The general lack of a 'thick description' may have been due to the study aims, or the choice of methods in which the studies were conducted.

4.10.4 Confidence in the findings of the review

As described in the methods section, we used the CERQual approach to assess the confidence of each review finding, grading each finding as either of high, moderate or low confidence. We assessed most of the findings as of moderate confidence because of the methodological limitations of the underlying studies. We assessed one study to be of low confidence because of concerns regarding both methodological limitations and adequacy with limited data. In this review, twenty-one (21) statements were generated and summarized into four (4) themes: potential facilitators of HIVST uptake, perceived barriers to HIVST, concerns about HIVST and HIVST experiences. The confidence in the findings of the review is summarized in Table 4.3.

4.11 Potential facilitators of HIVST uptake

Availability of HIVST

HIV experts, HIV policymakers and HIV care providers perceived the availability of HIVST as a factor would increase uptake of HIV testing, enable repeat testing, identifying first-time testers and early diagnosis, leading to the linkage of care and treatment. HIV care providers also identified availability of HIVST as an enabling factor.

> *"We need to look at all avenues so that people can access testing services at the moment [...], we think that the availability of self-testing in this country is going to help us to achieve that target (80%), [...]. The more clients repeat testing the more we can identify first-time testers and early diagnosis and more we can link to care and treatment. " [HIV policymaker].* (van Rooyen et al., 2015)

Stigma and discrimination associated with HIV testing

Furthermore, potential HIVST users identified the potential of HIVST to decrease stigma and discrimination associated with HIV testing, which will motivate men to uptake HIVST: *Men would accept [...] they would say, "aaah, why should the doctor test me? Aaah, it's better to be the first to know my HIV status." You would feel shy when meeting the doctor who knows that you are HIV positive* [Male, IDI].(Choko et al., 2017)

HIVST provides an opportunity to test for HIV

Participants agreed that HIVST provides an opportunity to test for HIV and to circumvent facility-based barriers, leading to increased uptake of self-testing: *Others have said it [HIVST] will alleviate the facility-related barriers-long waiting time, long queues and visibility by going to a centre or a mobile clinic. [Health care provider]*(Makusha et al., 2015).

HIVST and confidentiality of HIV test results

The possibility of HIVST to increase the confidentiality of HIV test results compared to conventional HIV testing approaches (i.e. voluntary counselling and testing, provider-initiated counselling and testing, mobile counselling and testing, etc.) were cited by participants.

> *"So I think the benefits of HIVST are pure confidentiality, if I can own the process myself, you know I would have that confidential aspect of HIV test results..." [HIV policy maker]*. (Makusha et al., 2015).

Perceived autonomy and self-empowerment

HIV experts, HIV policymakers, health care providers and potential HIVST users perceived that the autonomy to make one's own choice of HIV testing method and self- empowerment to take responsibility of one's life, including sexual health, is a potential facilitator to the uptake of HIVST. They believed that the perceived autonomy and self-empowerment would create a more active role of an individual in managing their health and decision-making process for HIV testing:

"...the self- empowerment to take responsibility for my life because if I can go as far as to decide that: "You know what, I need to be testing myself at this level", it means I am taking responsibility for my sexual health, [. .] [and] I am going to think about it in light of how I manage my life [HIV expert] (Makusha et al., 2015).

Perceived convenience of self-testing

Further, the convenience of self-testing (i.e. at home and/or any private place) in privacy was perceived as a potential facilitator. Participants believed that HIVST brings testing services closer to users and would attenuate travelling costs, waiting time at health facilities and save time for other income-generating activities, which will encourage uptake of HIV testing.

As a 28-year-old male participant explained:

"It is different from making the process of going to the clinic. Therefore, the number of people going to the clinic will decrease. And your daily budget, which you reserve, you will be able to buy the instrument because when you go to test at the clinic you incur costs like bus fare, eating and staying in queues. So those costs are reduced a bit " [28- year-old men, Non-tester] (Jennings et al., 2017).

Couple' HIVST and disclosure of HIV serostatus

HIV policymakers felt that HIVST might provide an opportunity for couples to talk before performing self-testing. They believed the face-to-face communication could facilitate the disclosure of HIV serostatus and hence reduce gender-based violence related to HIV positive results.

"[. . .] I see (HIVST) increasing couples' talking and in a way, we would probably reduce GBV [gender-based violence] because sometimes that's the problem. When one goes for a test and the other does not know and then the other one does find out, it is always detrimental" [HIV policy maker] (van Rooyen, Tulloch et al. 2015).

4.12 Potential barriers to HIVST

Affordability of HIVST kits

Affordability of HIVST kits was a recurring theme across the studies in this review. Potential HIVST users mentioned that the high cost of buying self-testing kits might hinder the uptake of HIV testing.

As a 28-year-old male participant explained:

"That's why I said that if it is sold at a lower price like from 15,000 to 20,000 [Tanzanian shillings ~$6.91 to $9.20] people will be able to buy it. But, if it will be sold at a higher price like at 30,000 to 40,000[Tanzanian shillings~$13.80 to $18.40], others will fail to buy it – as someone may have the ability to buy it, but says why should I buy it? But at a lower price, a person can buy it " [28-year-old-men, Non-tester]. (Jennings et al., 2017).

Perceived unreliability of self-test results

There was a commonly discussed belief among potential HIVST users on the unreliability of self-test results. They expressed their fear that the self-test kits may fail to accurately test for HIV. This fear came from their misconceptions about the presence of HIV in the blood sample and the misinterpretation of results when testing alone.

"So many people are not going for HIV test not because of the fear of the unknown but the fear that self-testing may fail to test accurately for HIV. Many people believe that HIV is in the blood...so taking a sample from the mouth to test for HIV and not a blood sample is the main reason for the fear"[Female Non-tester, IDI]. (Njau et al., 2014).

Low literacy and HIVST

Concern about low literacy particularly among people residing in rural settings was perceived as a potential barrier. Potential HIVST users believed that the inability to read might negatively influence the uptake of HIVST.

"Most people, particularly in the rural areas are illiterate; they can't read even a newspaper. How can they be able to read and follow the instructions of how to use the HIV self- testing kits?" [Male tester, IDI] (Njau et al., 2014).

Fear of a positive test result

One recurring theme across the studies included in this synthesis was the fear and anxiety of receiving a positive test result. For example, buying HIVST kits was compared with buying death or committing suicide. As a 26-year-old male participant explained:

"It is similar to buying death. It is like someone going to buy poison for committing suicide! So, I do not know whether the poison is right or wrong. The point of buying it is, as I said, buying my death. I mean just do not sell it. As none will buy it. If it is sold, it will be hard for someone to decide to go buy it. Trust me. You will go buy your death, I tell you" [26-year-old-men, Non-tester].(Jennings et al., 2017).

Perception about the low quality of HIVST kits

Beliefs about individual perceptions and previous experiences with fake medical equipment or low quality of HIVST kits and false advertisements were perceived as a major concern in this study. Most participants expressed their fear of the low quality of HIVST kits and false advertisements because of lack of poor quality assurance measures, which might undermine the uptake of HIVST:

[...] How will we ensure quality assurance and ensure that the manufacturers are not false advertising? How will we ensure that the self-tests are manufactured by an accredited facility? All these issues need to be addressed to provide a good regulatory system" [HIV policy maker].(Makusha et al., 2015).

4.13 Factors impending policy-maker adoption of HIVST intervention

HIV experts, HIV policymakers, health care providers and potential HIVST users expressed concerns related to HIVST. Such concerns included human rights issues, lack of linkage to HIV care and treatment, lack of face-to-face counselling, lack of regulatory and quality assurance systems and quality of HIVST kits.

Human rights issues

Human rights issues reported by most participants were based on how ethical HIVST is. Most participants considered HIVST ethical if it would provide more freedom, choices

However, HIVST may be unethical if it will increase, HIVST users/ vulnerabilities (i.e. coerced or forced testing) or used to limit their freedom and rights.

"[...] I can see lots of reluctance on the part of human rights people [...] It's more the human rights people, an instinct around coerced or forced testing. It is always about protecting the tiny percentage of people who are going to be abused." [HIV policymaker, South Africa].(van Rooyen et al., 2015).

Lack of linkage to HIV care and treatment

Another major concern expressed by HIV experts, HIV policymakers and health care providers was the lack of linkage to HIV care and treatment following a positive HIV result. They generally agreed that linkage to HIV care and treatment is an important component of HIVST and inextricably linked to counselling.

Additionally, they argued that HIVST should be regarded as a screening rather than a testing tool and put emphasis that a positive result needs to be followed by a confirmatory laboratory test at the health facility, which might facilitate linkage to HIV care and treatment.*"[. . .], there need to be clear instructions on how to get into care, what needs to be done if you test positive and if there could be a reliable helpline to call, that would be ideal so that people could seek confirmatory laboratory test at the health facility... [HIV expert].*(van Rooyen et al., 2015).

Lack of face-to-face counselling

Another concern about HIVST expressed by most participants was the lack of face-to-face counselling. They viewed counselling an essential component, which is missing in HIVST. From their perspective, lack of face-to-face counselling may increase the risk of psychopathic tendencies, suicidal ideation and coercion:

"Without adequate pre & post-test counselling, a reactive self-test result can lead to suicides, or murder, while some psychopaths may decide to embark on a 'revenge' vendetta by hiding their status and seeking opportunities for unprotected sex. Also, a negative result may encourage the individual to engage in irresponsible sexual activities"[HIV policy maker] (Makusha et al., 2015).

Lack of effective regulation of HIVST

HIV experts, HIV policymakers and health care providers perceived that lack of effective regulation of medicines and laboratory tests might jeopardize the uptake of HIVST because it would affect the quality assurance for HIVST kits.

Most agreed that regulatory and a quality assurance framework was essential for the uptake of HIVST.

> *[...] several issues in terms of laws and policies on medicines and related medical supplies need to be addressed. How will we ensure quality assurance and ensure that the manufacturers are not false advertising? How will we ensure that the self-tests are manufactured by an accredited facility? All these issues need to be*

4.14 HIV self-testing experiences

HIVST users believed that the availability of HIVST creates an opportunity for previous ART users to re-start treatment.

As explained by a female HIV positive participant:

"I was on ARVs [...], but [...] I stopped [....] I wanted to start again but was shouted at the hospital because I did not remember my number. This [HIVST] was a better way of re-starting taking ARVs" [Female, HIV positive, Discordant].(Kumwenda et al., 2014).

HIVST users believed that the ease of use of self-testing kits particularly with oral fluid-based HIV compared to finger stick/whole blood-based HIV testing could influence HIVST uptake. Further, most users expressed a preference for oral fluid-based HIV to finger stick/whole blood-based HIV. While most users reported ease of use of self-testing kits, user errors were common among self-testers. Few reported confusion on how to use self-test kits, because of lacking clear instructions on some steps on how to use the kits.

''[The step] was a bit confusing, because at first, I didn't know if I should remove it [cap] on the test or pour over it. No instructions were available for that step. Even the picture does not show.'' [Male tester] (Peck et al., 2014).

Finally, some self-testers reported their concern about the misinterpretation of test results because of different products of HIVST with different instructions on how to interpret results to increase rates of wrong interpretations of test results. As explained by a female HIVST user:

''Firstly we all know that if there are two lines it means it is positive so here there are two lines and they say it is invalid, for a villager they cannot understand this, it doesn't matter where the lines are but as long as there are two lines to many positive people, so they better look into that." [Female tester] (Peck et al., 2014).

4.15 Discussion

Overall, this synthesis highlighted a broad range of qualitative evidence on potential facilitators for and perceived barriers to uptake of HIVST from HIV experts, HIV policy-makers, health care providers and self-testing experiences of adult users in Africa.

The findings of this synthesis are important for understanding the wider array of factors that may facilitate or hinder HIVST uptake and HIVST experiences of adult users in Africa. The findings will also give an insight on how to integrate HIVST into the broader HIV testing services.

Our findings have implications for future studies assessing the feasibility of HIVST in Africa and provide valuable information for HIV stakeholders and interventionists to consider as they develop policy and/ or evaluate HIVST interventions.
Commonly cited potential facilitators of HIVST across the literature such as availability of HIVST, privacy and confidentiality, convenience and disclosure to sero status (Kebede et al., 2013, van Dyk 2013, Brown et al., 2015, Jennings et al., 2017, Knight et al., 2017), the ability of HIVST to decrease stigma and discrimination, the potential of HIVST to circumvent facility-based barriers, increase the confidentiality of HIV test results after self-testing and, perceived autonomy and self-empowerment in decision-making to test were also found amongst participants in this synthesis (Makusha et al., 2015, van Rooyen et al., 2015, Harichund and Moshabela 2017).

In this synthesis, high costs of HIVST test kits, the unreliability of self-testing results, low literacy and fear and anxiety of positive test results, may mitigate effective HIVST uptake in different settings in Africa. These findings are consistent with existing literature on potential barriers to HIVST globally (Brown et al., 2015, Kurth et al., 2016, Harichund and Moshabela 2017). For example, there are different views regarding the cost of HIVST kits across sub-regions of Africa. Since most countries in Africa are resource-poor, most participants felt that HIVST should be free of charge subsidized by the government, similar to the current conventional HIV testing approaches (Jennings et al., 2017, Knight et al., 2017). In other settings, assurance of privacy and confidentiality at distribution points for delivery of self-test kits influence some participants' willingness to pay for HIVST kits (Brown et al., 2015, van Rooyen et al., 2015, Maheswaran et al., 2016, Knight et al., 2017). However, there is a gap in the literature on how to achieve free of charge HIVST kits in the for-profit context and calls for empirical research to fill this gap (Gagnon et al., 2018).

The findings from this synthesis highlight that the perceived inability of self-test kits to accurately test for HIV and the misinterpretation of test results may undermine the uptake of HIVST test kits. Participants across studies included in this synthesis agreed that information on how rapid HIV tests function may alleviate misconceptions, thus improving the uptake of testing (Makusha et al., 2015, van Rooyen et al., 2015).

Irrespective of existing global evidence on potential benefits of HIVST (Njau et al., 2014, Brown et al., 2015, Makusha et al., 2015, van Rooyen et al., 2015, Choko et al., 2017, Indravudh et al., 2017, Jennings et al., 2017, Knight et al., 2017), participants in this synthesis expressed key concerns related to HIVST. The concerns include human rights issues, lack of regulatory and quality assurance systems, low quality of HIVST kits, lack

These findings align with existing literature on concerns related to HIVST, such as regulation. For example, Johnson and colleagues (Johnson et al., 2014), agreed that state regulation was an essential requirement to achieve quality assurance and hence promote quality of HIVST kits to the advantage of the users. However, caution was raised regarding state regulation to restrict access to HIVST, such as setting an age limit for purchasing test kits, because the purchase of an HIVST kit was a personal decision that should not be interfered by the state (Allais and Venter 2014, Hurt and Powers 2014, Scott 2014, Gagnon et al., 2018). Therefore, it behoves HIV policymakers and interventionists to develop country-specific HIVST regulatory and policy frameworks that focus on safety, prevention of coercive use and effectiveness of HIVST (Ganguli et al., 2009, Mavedzenge et al., 2013, Wong et al., 2014).

To address the potential lack of linkage to care and face-to-face counselling, this synthesis recommends innovative counselling and training approaches for users of HIVST. Strategies to increase linkage to HIV prevention, care and treatment after HIVST include home visits or phone calls (Chipungu et al., 2017) and demand-side financial incentives (Choko et al., 2018). Strategies such as the use of toll-free phone numbers provided by the manufacturers of HIVST for counselling have been perceived of greater quality than face-to-face counselling in different settings (Arnold 2012, Figueroa et al., 2015).

Further, there is a need for research to evaluate algorithms and methods that will facilitate adequate linkage to care following HIVST (Ganguli et al., 2009, Mavedzenge et al., 2013, Wong et al., 2014). However, Gagnon et al. (2018) caution that such strategies could indirectly propagate stigma by making HIV testing a "clandestine activity" done in secrecy in home settings.

This synthesis identified two qualitative studies reporting self-testing experiences among adult men and women in Kenya, Malawi and South Africa (Kumwenda et al., 2014, Peck et al., 2014). Participants reported that the availability of HIVST created an opportunity for re-initiation of ART, suggesting that defaulters may be more likely to prefer HIVST than standard HTS to re-initiate HIV care and treatment.

Easy to use of HIVST kits and preference of oral fluid-based HIV rapid test (RDT) because it is less invasive and painless was frequently mentioned by HIVST users. These findings align with existing literature on HIVST, suggesting that most users (even with low literacy) find HIVST is easy to use (Ochako et al., 2014) and may prefer oral fluid-based HIV RDT to finger stick or whole blood-based HIV testing (Gaydos et al., 2011, Peck et al., 2014, Figueroa et al., 2015).

Confusion on how to use HIVST kits was the main cause of user errors and inaccuracy, particularly with unsupervised HIVST (Peck et al 2014) and concurs with findings

The observation underlines the need to provide training on HIVST use, accompanied with clear pictorial instructions-for-use in local language on how to perform HIVST, easy steps to interpret the test result and linkage to support and counselling services (Lee et al., 2007, Ng et al., 2012, Figueroa et al., 2015, Ortblad et al., 2018).

Moreover, different products of HIVST kits with different manufacturers' instructions might increase risks of wrong interpretation of test results. In considering, new HIVST products, which are under development and could be adapted for HIVST, manufacturers should be cautioned to develop user-friendly HIVST products to reduce user errors (Makusha et al., 2015, van Rooyen et al., 2015).

4.15.1 Strengths and limitation

The strength of this synthesis is the systematic search of multiple databases to identify all relevant qualitative studies meeting the pre-defined inclusion criteria. Additionally, we included studies using different methodological approaches, contributing to the in-depth understanding of HIV stakeholders' perceptions of the factors that enable or deter the uptake of HIV self-testing in Africa. Including studies conducted among actual users of HIVST was another strength, because they provided findings relevant to the research question, as opposed to studies conducted on hypothetical use of HIVST.

Studies with overall 'low quality' were not excluded if they added pertinent qualitative evidence. This resulted in a comprehensive review encapsulating a range of perspectives related to the study objectives. Another strength was the use of the CASP tool for methodological quality assessment (CASP 2014), and *CERQual*, for the confidence of qualitative evidence (Lewin et al., 2018).
The use of these multiple approaches had advantages, including the possibility to reach conclusions based on similarities identified in heterogeneous studies, more accessibility to a wider audience than primary studies and providing a weight of evidence about HIVST.

There are however some limitations of this synthesis. Foremost, the possibility that this review might not reflect all the barriers, facilitators and actual users' experiences related to HIVST that are relevant could be a limitation because of the few studies conducted across African countries. Seven primary studies reported views of HIV stakeholders about the hypothetical use of HIVST, which may not reflect their actual practice. Only two primary studies reported the actual practice of self-testing among adult users, indicating a need for further research on HIVST testing experiences across different

A second limitation is the possibility of missing some publications. To mitigate this limitation, we scanned references of selected papers for additional studies. Because of language restraints, we only included papers published in English and the findings reported henceforth may be subject to English language publication bias.

4.16 Conclusions

Generally, the uptake of HIV testing in Africa is a complex process influenced by multifaceted and interlinked factors. This synthesis contributed to a literature gap on HIVST by identifying important factors that enable or deter the uptake of HIVST among adults in Africa. While identified facilitators of and barriers to the uptake of HIVST cut across studies from sub-regions of Africa, HIVST interventionists should develop context-specific, culturally appropriate strategies to increase uptake of HIV testing using HIVST. Actual HIVST users expressed preference for oral-fluid self-testing because it is easy to use, less invasive and painless compared to finger-stick/whole blood-based HIV tests. Lack of clear instructions on how to use self-test kits and existing different products of HIVST increases user errors. If adopted as a complimentary HTS option, HIVST could facilitate early detection, early care, treatment and prevention and maybe pivotal in providing an invaluable tool to increase access to HIV care, treatment and prevention to achieve the 95-95-95 by 2030 (UNAIDS 2017, UNAIDS 2018, UNAIDS 2019).

References

Allais, L. and F. Venter (2014). "The Ethical, Legal and Human Rights Concerns Raised by Licensing HIV Self-Testing for Private Use." AIDS Behaviour **18**(4): 433-437.

Arnold, C. (2012). "At-home HIV test poses dilemmas and opportunities." Lancet **380**(9847): 1045-1046.

Barnett-Page, E. and J. Thomas (Effective Practice and Organisation of Care 2009). "Methods for the synthesis of qualitative research: a critical review." BMC Medical Research Methodology **9**: 59.

Britten, N., R. Campbell, C. Pope, J. Donovan, M. Morgan and R. Pill (2002). "Using meta-ethnography to synthesize qualitative research: a worked example." Journal of Health Services Research and Policy **7**: 209-215.

Brown, B., M. O. Folayan, A. Imosili, F. Durueke and A. Amuamuziam (2015). "HIV self-testing in Nigeria: Public opinions and perspectives." Global public health **10**(3): 354-365.

Campbell, R., P. Pound, M. Morgan, G. Daker-White, N. Britten, R. Pill, et al. (2003). "Evaluating meta-ethnography: systematic analysis and synthesis of qualitative research." Social Science & Medicine **56**(4): 671-684.

CASP. (2014). "Critical Appraisal Skills Programme qualitative research checklist 31.05.13.". from ÂČČÆĖĔÅ ZYÃVĬĔÃĐĬXĄÅ ĖĊÁYĖYYZYĬĨĠĬİ X.

Chipungu, J., S. Bosomprah, A. Zanolini, H. Thimurthy, R. Chilengi, A. Sharma, et al. (2017). "Understanding linkage to care with HIV self-test approach in Lusaka, Zambia - A mixed-method approach " PLoS ONE **12**(11): e0187998

Choko, A., S. Candfield, H. Maheswaran, A. Lepine, E. L. Corbett and K. Fielding (2018). "The effect of demand-side financial incentives for increasing linkage into HIV treatment and voluntary medical male circumcision: A systematic review and meta-analysis of randomized controlled trials in low- and middle-income countries." PLoS ONE **13**(11): e0207263.

Choko, A. T., N. Desmond, E. L. Webb, K. Chavula, S. Napierala-Mavedzenge, C. A. Gaydos, et al. (2011). "The Uptake and Accuracy of Oral Kits for HIV Self-Testing in High HIV Prevalence Setting: A Cross-Sectional Feasibility Study in Blantyre, Malawi." PLoS Medicine **8**(Critical Appraisal Skills Programme 2010).

Choko, A. T., M. K. Kumwenda, C. C. Johnson, D. W. Sakala, M. C. Chikalipo, K. Fielding, et al. (2017). "Acceptability of woman-delivered HIV self-testing to the male partner and additional interventions: a qualitative study of antenatal care participants in Malawi." Journal of the International Aids Society **20**(1): 1-10.

Colvin, C. J., R. Garside, M. Wainwright, H. Munthe-Kaas, C. Glenton, M. A. Bohren, et al. (2018). "Applying GRADE-CERQual to qualitative evidence synthesis findings-paper 4: how to assess coherence." Implementation Science **13**(Suppl 1): 13.

Figueroa, C., C. Johnson, A. Verster and R. Baggaley (2015). "Attitudes and Acceptability on HIV Self-testing Among Key Populations: A Literature Review." AIDS and Behavior: 1-17.

Gagnon, M., M. French and Y. Hebert (2018). "The HIV self-testing debate: where do we stand?" BMC Int Health Hum Rights **18**(1): 5.

Ganguli, I., I. V. Bassett, K. L. Dong and R. P. Walensky (Effective Practice and Organisation of Care 2009). "Home testing for HIV infection in resource-limited settings." Current HIV/AIDS Report (Critical Appraisal Skills Programme 2010) 7:77–84 **6**(4): 217-223.

Gaydos, C. A., Y. H. Hsieh, L. Harvey, A. Burah and H. Won, et al. (2011). "Will patients "opt-in" to perform their own rapid HIV test in the emergency departments?" Annals of Emergency Medicine **58**: S74-78.

Glenton, C., B. Carlsen, S. Lewin, H. Munthe-Kaas, C. J. Colvin, O. Tuncalp, et al. (2018). "Applying GRADE-CERQual to qualitative evidence synthesis findings-paper 5: how to assess the adequacy of data." Implement Sci **13**(Suppl 1): 14.

Harichund, C. and M. Moshabela (2017). "Acceptability of HIV Self-Testing in Sub-Saharan Africa: Scoping Study." AIDS Behavior **22**: 560-568.

Hurt, C. B. and K. A. Powers (2014). "Self-testing for HIV and its impact on public health." Sexually Transmitted Diseases **41**(1): 10-12.

Indravudh, P. P., E. L. Sibanda, M. d'Elbee, M. K. Kumwenda, B. Ringwald, G. Maringwa, et al. (2017). "'I will choose when to test, where I want to test': investigating young people's preferences for HIV self-testing in Malawi and Zimbabwe." AIDS **31 Suppl 3**: S203-S212.

Jennings, L., D. F. Conserve, J. Merrill, L. Kajula, J. Iwelunmor, S. Linnemayr, et al. (2017). "Perceived Cost Advantages and Disadvantages of Purchasing HIV Self- Testing Kits among Urban Tanzanian Men: An Inductive Content Analysis." Journal of AIDS & Clinical Research **08**(08).

Johnson, C., R. Baggaley, S. Forsythe, H. van Rooyen, N. Ford, S. Napierala Mavedzenge, et al. (2014). "Realizing the Potential for HIV Self-Testing." AIDS Behavior.

Johnson, C. C., C. Kennedy, V. A. Fonner, N. Siegfried, C. Figueroa, S. Dalal, et al. (2017). "Examining

Kebede, B., T. Abate and D. Mekonnen (2013). "HIV self-testing practices among Health care Workers: feasibility and options for accelerating HIV testing services in Ethiopia." Pan African Medical Journal **15**(50): 1-8.

Knight, L., T. Makusha, J. Lim, R. Peck, M. Taegtmeyer and H. van Rooyen (2017). "I think it is right": a qualitative exploration of the acceptability and desired future use of oral swab and finger-prick HIV self-tests by lay users in KwaZulu-Natal, South Africa." BMC Research Notes **10**(1): 486.

Krause, J., F. Subklew-Sehume, C. Kenyon and R. Colebunders (2013). "Acceptability of HIV self-testing: a systematic literature review." BMC Public Health **13:**(735.): 1-19.

Kumwenda, M., A. Munthali, M. Phiri, D. Mwale, T. Gutteberg, E. MacPherson, et al. (2014). "Factors shaping initial decision-making to self-test amongst cohabiting couples in urban Blantyre, Malawi." AIDS Behavior **18 Suppl 4**: S396-404.

Kurth, A. E., C. M. Cleland, N. Chhun, J. E. Sidle, E. Were, V. Naanyu, et al. (2016). "Accuracy and Acceptability of Oral Fluid HIV Self-Testing in a General Adult Population in Kenya." AIDS Behavior **20**(4): 870-879.

Lee, V. J., S. C. Tan, A. Earnest, P. S. Seong, H. H. Tan and Y. S. Leo (2007). "User acceptability and feasibility of self-testing with HIV rapid tests." Journal of Acquired Immune Deficiency Syndromes **45**(4): 449-453.

Lewin, S., A. Booth, C. Glenton, H. Munthe-Kaas, A. Rashidian, M. Wainwright, et al. (2018). "Applying GRADE-CERQual to qualitative evidence synthesis findings: introduction to the series." Implementation Science **13**(S1).

Lewin, S., C. Glenton, H. Munthe-Kaas, B. Carlsen, C. J. Colvin, M. Gulmezoglu, et al. (2015). "Using qualitative evidence in decision making for health and social interventions: an approach to assess confidence in findings from qualitative evidence syntheses (GRADE-CERQual)." PLoS Medicine **12**(Critical Appraisal Skills Programme 2010): e1001895.

Maheswaran, H., S. Petrou, P. MacPherson, A. T. Choko, F. Kumwenda, D. G. Lalloo, et al. (2016). "Cost and quality of life analysis of HIV self-testing and facility-based HIV testing and counselling in Blantyre, Malawi." BMC Medicine **14**: 34.

Makusha, T., L. Knight, M. Taegtmeyer, O. Tulloch, A. Davids, J. Lim, et al. (2015). "HIV Self-Testing Could "Revolutionize Testing in South Africa, but It Has Got to Be Done Properly": Perceptions of Key Stakeholders." PLoS ONE **10**(3): e0122783.

Mavedzenge, S., R. Baggaley and E. A. Corbett (2013). "Review of self-testing for HIV: research and policy priorities in a new era of HIV prevention." Clinical Infectious Diseases **57**(1): 126-138.

Merten, S., E. Kenter, O. McKenzie, M. Musheke, H. Ntalasha and A. Martin-Hilber (Critical Appraisal Skills Programme 2010). "Patient-reported barriers and drivers of adherence to antiretrovirals in sub-Saharan Africa: a meta-ethnography." Tropical Medicine & International Health **15 Suppl 1**: 16-33.

Munthe-Kaas, H., M. A. Bohren, C. Glenton, S. Lewin, J. Noyes, O. Tuncalp, et al. (2018). "Applying GRADE-CERQual to qualitative evidence synthesis findings-paper 3: how to assess methodological limitations." Implementation Science **13**(Suppl 1): 9.

Ng, O. T., A. L. Chow, V. J. Lee, M. I. C. Chen, M. K. Win, H. H. Tan, et al. (2012). "Accuracy and User-Acceptability of HIV Self-Testing Using an Oral fluid-based HIV Rapid Test." PLoS ONE 7(Effective Practice and Organisation of Care 2009): e45168. Doi:10.1371/journal.pone.0045168.

Njau, B., J. Ostermann, D. Brown, A. Muhlbacher, E. Reddy and N. Thielman (2014). "HIV testing

Noyes, J., A. Booth, S. Lewin, B. Carlsen, C. Glenton, C. J. Colvin, et al. (2018). "Applying GRADE-CERQual to qualitative evidence synthesis findings-paper 6: how to assess the relevance of the data." Implementation Science **13**(Suppl 1): 4.

Noyes, J., J. Popay, A. Pearson, K. Hannes and A. Booth (Effective Practice and Organisation of Care 2009). Chapter 20: Qualitative research and Cochrane reviews.In: Higgins JPT, Green S editor(s). Cochrane Handbook of Systematic Reviews for Interventions Version 5.0.2[updated 2009].

Ochako, R., L. Vu and K. Peterson (2014). Insights Into Potential Users and Messaging for HIV Oral Self-Test Kits in Kenya. Washington, DC, International Initiative for Impact Evaluation.

Orasure. (2017). "OraQuick HIV Self-test." from ÂČČÆĖĖĎĎĎ ĄĆVĈĆZÆĄÅĖÆĆĄĊXĈĒÆÀÆČĄĊĈĒ ĄĆVÆÆÆĈÆÆÆĈÆĈÆ

Ortblad, K. F., D. Kibuuka Musoke, T. Ngabirano, A. Nakitende, G. Taasi, L. G. Barresi, et al. (2018). "HIV self-test performance among female sex workers in Kampala, Uganda: a cross-sectional study." BMJ Open **8**(11): e022652.

Pai, N. P., J. Sharma, S. Shivkumar, S. Pillay, C. Vadnais, L. Joseph, et al. (2013). "Supervised and Unsupervised Self-Testing for HIV in High- and Low-Risk Populations: A Systematic Review." PLoS Medicine **10(4):** : e1001414. .

Peck, R. B., J. M. Lim, H. van Rooyen, W. Mukoma, L. Chepuka, P. Bansil, et al. (2014). "What should the ideal HIV self-test look like? A usability study of test prototypes in unsupervised HIV self-testing in Kenya, Malawi and South Africa." AIDS Behavior **18 Suppl 4**: S422-432.

Scott, P. A. (2014). "Unsupervised self-testing as part of public health screening for HIV in resource-poor environments: some ethical considerations." AIDS Behaviour **18 Suppl 4**: S438-444.

Suthar, A. B., N. Ford, P. J. Bachanas, V. J. Wong, J. S. Rajan, A. K. Saltzman, et al. (2013). "Towards Universal Voluntary HIV Testing and Counselling: A Systematic Review and Meta-Analysis of Community-Based Approaches." PLoS Medicine **10(8):**(e1001496.).

Thomas, J. and A. Harden (2008). "Methods for the thematic synthesis of qualitative research in systematic reviews." BMC Medical Research Methodology **8**: 45.

Tonen-Wolyec, S., S. Batina-Agasa, J. Muwonga, F. Fwamba N'kulu, R. S. Mboumba Bouassa and L. Belec (2018). "Evaluation of the practicability and virological performance of finger-stick whole-blood HIV self-testing in French-speaking sub-Saharan Africa." PLoS ONE **13**(1): e0189475.

Tong, A., K. Flemming, E. McInnes, S. Oliver and J. Craig (2012). "Enhancing transparency in reporting the synthesis of qualitative research: ENTREQ." BMC Medical Research Methodology.

UNAIDS (2017). "UNAIDS Data ".

UNAIDS. (2018). Global AIDS Update 2018: Miles To Go Closing Gaps Breaking Barriers Righting Injustices.

van Dyk, A. C. (2013). "Client-initiated, provider-initiated, or self-testing for HIV: what do South Africans prefer?" Journal of Association of Nurses AIDS Care **24**(6): e45-56.

van Rooyen, H., O. Tulloch, W. Mukoma, T. Makusha, L. Chepuka, L. C. Knight, et al. (2015). "What are the constraints and opportunities for HIVST scale-up in Africa? Evidence from Kenya, Malawi and South Africa." Journal of the International Aids Society **18**(1): 19445.

Wong, V., E. Jenkins, N. Ford and H. Ingold (2019). "To thine own test be true: HIV self - testing and the global reach for the undiagnosed." Journal of the International Aids Society **22**(S1): e25256.

W. H. O. (2015). WHO prequalification: Sample product dossier for an IVD intended for HIV self-testing. SIMUTM self-test for HIV 12O working document, December 2015.

W. H. O. (2015). WHO prequalification: Sample product dossier for an IVD intended for HIV self-testing. SIMUTM self-test for HIV 12O working document.

Wun, H., D. Kang, T. Huang, Y. Qian, X. Li, E. C. Wilson, et al. (2013). "Factors Associated with Willingness to Accept Oral Fluid HIV rapid Testing among Most-at-Risk Populations in China." PLoS ONE **8**(11): e80594.

CHAPTER FIVE

5.0 Acceptability of HIV Self-Testing: A formative qualitative study among individuals, community and HIV testing experts in Northern Tanzania.

5.1 Introduction

In 2018, an estimated 37.9 million people were living with HIV worldwide, 770,000 died of HIV related diseases and nearly 40 % of adults were unaware of their HIV status (UNAIDS 2017, UNAIDS 2019). HIV /AIDS is a leading cause of death among Tanzanians, with an estimated 80,000 deaths annually. By 2017, an estimated 1.5 million people were living with HIV and 83,000 are newly infected each year (UNAIDS 2017, UNAIDS 2019).

Evidence has shown that HIV testing services (HTS) is an essential component of HIV/AIDS control programmes globally and an entry point of the HIV testing cascade. Major benefits associated with HTS include early detection, early initiation of treatment and care and the introduction of risk reduction strategies for HIV acquisition or onward transmission (UNAIDS/WHO 2010, Wanyenze et al., 2011, UNAIDS 2015, UNAIDS 2017, UNAIDS 2019).

In Tanzania, HTS are available in more than 2,000 sites, including facility-based approaches, which are the most common. Other HTS options, including home-based, mobile or outreach testing campaigns available at venues such as schools, markets, workplaces, have been occasionally implemented with significant success (United Republic of Tanzania National Bureau of Statistics and ICF 2013). Additionally, the Tanzanian Ministry of Health and Social Welfare (MoHSW) in 2007 developed guidelines for HTS in clinical settings to complement the client-initiated testing which had failed to capture important patient groups (United Republic of Tanzania and Ministry of Health and Social Welfare National Aids Control Programme 2007).

Despite the benefits of HTS and the widespread availability of varied HTS options, availability of ART for people living with HIV testing rates remains low in Tanzania. According to the 2016-2017 Tanzania HIV Indicator Survey (THIS), 44.1 % of women and 54. 7 % of men aged 15-64 years have never been tested for HIV. Additionally, only 30% of women and 25 % of men tested and received their results in the past year (THIS 2017).
In the Kilimanjaro region, public health officials have identified two high-risk populations: female bar workers (FBWs) and mountain climbing porters (MCPs).

Based on the 2013 Moshi municipal alcohol beverage licensing data, it is estimated that 2,000 young women between the ages of 18 and 40 years are working in more than 600 licensed establishments, with additional FBWs working in unlicensed alcohol selling venues. In both licensed and unlicensed venues, FBW have no permanent employment and are paid low wages e.g. Tanzanian Shillings (TZS) 80,000/= per month (US$ 1= 2,000 TZS).

There is evidence of 19 % to 26% HIV prevalence among FBWs, compared to 5.1 % HIV prevalence in the general population (THIS 2017). The observed high HIV prevalence among FBWs is associated with HIV risk behaviours, such as excessive alcohol consumption, multiple sexual partnerships and transactional sexual practices (Kapiga et al., 2002, A et al., 2006). Evidence suggests that less than 5% of FBWs have never tested for HIV, but 41% of those who have tested have never repeated HIV testing in the past year (Ostermann et al., 2015).

An estimated 17,000 porters working in the tourist industry are between the ages of 18 and 45 years, but are predominantly young men who are very mobile and face volatile income cycles (Peaty 2010). During high season (i.e., January to March and June to October), MCPs spend an extended time away from home supporting climbers of Mt. Kilimanjaro. For example, a trip to the top of the Mt. Kilimanjaro takes a minimum of 7 to 10 days depending on the route and the weather. A MCP can climb up to three trips non-stop per month for a total of 30 days. A descriptive cross-sectional study among MCPs showed behavioural risk factors for HIV infection, including unprotected sex, multiple concurrent sexual partnerships and substance use, including excessive alcohol consumption and marijuana use, suggesting a need to motivate sexually active MCPs to engage in HIV prevention interventions (Lyamuya et al., 2017). Further, one-third of MCPs have never tested for HIV, despite engaging in high-risk behaviours for HIV infection (Ostermann et al., 2015).

Previous studies have documented barriers to accessing HTS in clinical settings, which include stigma and discrimination related to HIV positive results (Mukolo et al., 2013, Njau et al., 2014, Ostermann et al., 2014). Other barriers are fear of visibility and lack of confidentiality of HIV positive test results (Mukolo et al., 2013), a lack of privacy and long waiting time to obtain a test result (Musheke et al., 2013).

HIV self-testing (HIVST) has the potential to circumvent these barriers to reach high-risk individuals in the population (Pai et al., 2013, WHO 2016, Johnson et al., 2017). HIVST refers specifically to a process in which an individual collects his or her specimen (oral

Multiple benefits have been documented that facilitate the high acceptability of HIVST among different target populations (Pai et al., 2013). Commonly cited benefits include convenience to test at home, privacy and confidentiality (Johnson et al., 2014), reduction of stigma due to less visibility (Kumwenda et al., 2014) and lower direct and indirect costs compared with going to an HIV testing point (Maheswaran et al., 2016). Also, the features of HIVST that have been regarded as benefits are that it is easy to use, results are obtained in a short time, it is painless and the non-invasive nature of oral-fluid tests (Xun et al., 2013). HIVST has shown the potential for reaching high-risk populations, including young people and enabling them to know their sero status (Johnson et al., 2014, Johnson et al., 2017).

In 2012, the US Food and Drug Administration approved an oral HIV self-test: Oral Quick available over-the-counter for HIV self-testing (US Food and Drug Administration(FDA) 2012). The approval of the HIVST sparked self-testing initiatives, particularly in high-income countries, with few studies from low- and middle-income countries (LMICs). To support the self-testing initiatives, the WHO developed guidelines for HIVST and partner notification, indicating that HIVST should be recommended as an additional testing option to the existing HTS (WHO 2016).

The purpose of this qualitative research was to inform the design of a behaviour change intervention (BCI) for FBWs and MCPs in Northern Tanzania. In preparation for the development of the BCI, we conducted in-depth interviews (IDIs) among key informants to understand their knowledge about the motivation and beliefs of the community towards HIVST uptake and linkage to HIV prevention, care and treatment, and focus group discussions (FGDs) among FBWs and MCPs to explore their beliefs, attitudes and personal agency towards HIVST uptake. In this study, key informants are defined as a group of community experts including HIV experts, HTS counsellors, community leaders and clinicians- who have particular knowledge and understanding of the community in the study setting.

5.2 Methods

5.2.1 Theoretical paradigm

The IBM was adopted in this study because it includes constructs from other influential behaviour theories such as the Theory of Reasoned Action (TRA), the Theory of Planned Behavior (TPB), Social Cognitive Theory (SCT) and the Health Belief Model (HBM). All these theories emphasize that value and expectancy beliefs guide behaviour (Fishbein and Azjen 1975, Godin and Kok 1996, Baranowski et al., 2002, Fishbein and Cappella 2006, Montaño et al., 2014).

Existing evidence suggests that the IBM framework focuses on determinants associated with HIV prevention behaviours, such as HIV testing (Kakoko et al., 2006, Mirkuzie et al., 2011, Abamecha et al., 2013, Montaño et al., 2014).

The Integrated Behavior Model (IBM) was used to identify the key specific beliefs that best explain MCPs' and FBWs' attitudes, perceived norms and personal agency towards HIVST. The IBM is composed of three key constructs, which are (a) attitude towards the behaviour (b) perceived norms and (c) personal agency (Glanz et al., 2008). The IBM further categorizes attitude into two components (a) experiential, which refers to a person's emotional reaction to the idea of performing the behaviour and (b) instrumental, which is defined as an individual's belief about the anticipated positive or negative consequences related to the recommended behaviour (Fishbein and Cappella 2006).

The construct "perceived norm" is categorized into two components (a) injunctive norm and (b) descriptive norm. An injunctive norm refers to an individual's belief about the extent to which significant others expect them to do or not to do the recommended behaviour. A descriptive norm refers to an individual's perception about what peers or relatives (i.e. parents, spouses, relatives, religious leaders, etc.) do regarding the recommended behaviour (Baranowski et al., 2002). Finally, the construct personal agency is also categorized into two components: (a) self-efficacy and (b) perceived control. Self-efficacy is the confidence an individual has about his or her capacity to perform the desired behaviour, while perceived control refers to an individual's perceived likelihood of occurrence of each facilitating or constraining condition and beliefs about the effect of facilitators and barriers to behavioural performance (Baranowski et al., 2002, Bandura 2004, Glanz et al., 2008). The IBM postulates that a person's intention to perform a behaviour and ultimately the performance of the behaviour (e.g. HIVST) is influenced by their attitudes, perceived norms and personal agency (Glanz et al., 2008). Figure 5.1 overleaf.

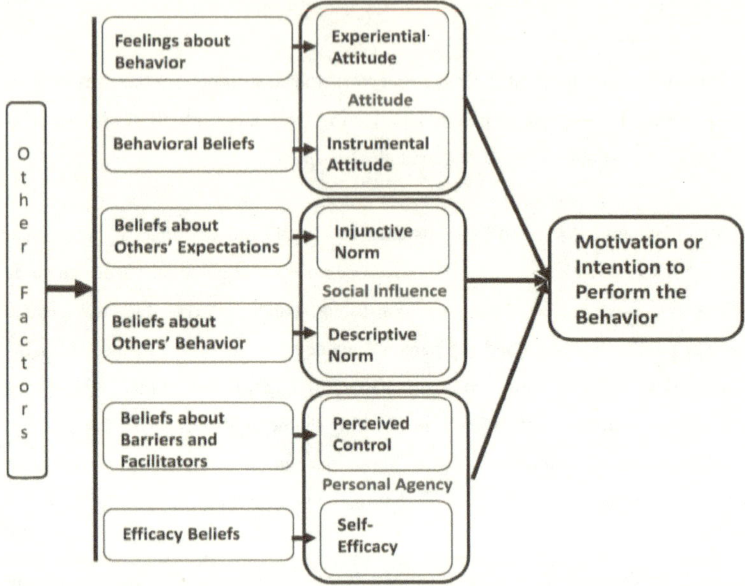

Figure 5.1. Integrated Behavior Model (adapted from Glanz, et al., 2008).

The study used the IBM to explore FBWs' and MCPs' attitudes, perceived norms and beliefs about personal agency related to HIVST uptake. The expected findings would inform the development of a BCI to increase HIVST uptake and linkage to HIV prevention, care and treatment for these populations.

5.3 Study Design and setting

This qualitative formative study was conducted between February 2017 and August 2017 in an urban setting in northern Tanzania with an estimated population of 202,379 inhabitants (United Republic of Tanzania 2012). Urban Moshi covers 59 square kilometres (23 sq. m) and is one of the seven administrative districts of Kilimanjaro region. The tribal groupings residing in the study area are the Chagaa and Pare. The main language used in the study setting is the national language, Kiswahili, spoken by most Tanzanians. The study area is on the tourist circuit, including bars, tourist hotels, major national parks and the highest mountain in Africa, Mt. Kilimanjaro.

At the time of the study, there were 51 health facilities in Moshi urban, which included hospitals (n=3), health centres (n=6), dispensaries (n= 14) and freestanding VCT facilities (n=2). Of these health facilities, 17 were public, 3 private/for-profits, 3 faith-based organizations and 2 non-governmental organizations. Besides, eight HIV Care and Treatment Centres (CTCs) provided access to confirmatory test and antiretroviral therapy for clients who tested HIV positive (Ostermann et al., 2014).

In 2007 and 2008, a nationwide HIV testing campaign attracted more than 24,000 testers in the study area (United Republic of Tanzania National Bureau of Statistics and ICF 2013).

5.3.1 Study population

The study populations were key informants (KIs), including HIV experts, HTS counsellors, community leaders, clinicians and MCPs and FBWs.

5.3.2 Sampling and Consenting

We conducted in-depth interviews (IDIs) with KI described in 5.3.1 above. Purposive sampling (Singleton and Straits 2005) was employed to recruit 18 KIs as IDI participants (male = 12; females = 6), with varying socio-demographic characteristics (e.g. sex, age, occupation, education, marital status, HIV testing experiences, etc.). The sampling approach was chosen to ensure the inclusion of a variety of viewpoints and diverse experiences among participants. HIV experts were recruited at their respective workplaces. Clinicians were recruited from public and private health facilities and influential leaders were recruited through local government structures. Subsequently, we conducted focus group discussions (FGDs) with MCPs and FBWs, some of whom had previously been tested for HIV and others who had never been tested. First, we obtained a list of alcoholic beverage license holders from the Moshi municipal council. Research assistants (RAs) visited each establishment and ascertained the number of FBWs who worked at each establishment and their shift schedules. The RAs offered invitation cards with contact information to eligible FBWs to visit the study's research office to undergo informed consent and participate in the study. A list of tour companies located in the study setting was obtained from the Moshi municipal council. The RAs visited all existing tourist companies and obtained information on the number of MCPs to get the actual number of all porters. The invitation process was the same as for FBWs (Ostermann et al., 2015).

In the sampling, FGD participants were recruited through door-to-door contact from randomly selected bars and tourist companies in urban Moshi. Participants were stratified by gender and HIV testing status (previously tested for HIV vs. never tested for HIV) and aimed at having between 6 and 12 participants per FGD. In total 37 (MCPs=21; FBWs=16) people participated in four FGDs, with 6 to 12 participants per group. All participants were 18 years old and above and able to provide consent. Participants were informed that participation in the study was voluntary and that they were free to withdraw at any point. Participants were assigned numbers to ensure anonymity and confidentiality and no personal identifiers were included in the collected data.

5.3.3 Focus group discussions and in-depth interviews

All FGDs and IDIs were conducted in Kiswahili - the national language spoken by most

Interview guide for IDIs was adopted from a previous qualitative study and for FGDs were based on the IBM constructs (Appendix F & G).

First, IDIs with KIs was used to explore their knowledge about the motivation and beliefs of the community on HIVST. FGDs were subsequently conducted with MCPs and FBWs to explore their attitudes, perceived norms and beliefs about personal agency related to HIVST uptake.

Sample interview guide questions for FGDs related to the IBM constructs included:-

1. Experiential attitudes: *"How do you feel about the idea of HIVST?"*
2. Instrumental attitudes: *"What are the negative/ or positive consequences that might result from you doing HVST?"*
3. Injunctive norms: "*What would people who are important to you (e.g. parents, spouses, relatives, peers, religious leaders, etc.) think you should do regarding HIVST?"*
4. Descriptive norms: *"What would people who are important to you (e.g. parents, spouses, relatives, peers, religious leaders, etc.) do about HIVST?"*
5. Perceived control: *"What do you think will make it easy or hard for you to do HIVST?"*

ÏË Self-efficacy: *"How confident are you that you would self-test for HIV?"*

IDIs were conducted at the respective enrolment venues of KIs (i.e. workplaces, public/private health facilities and local administrative structures, etc.), which lasted approximately 45 minutes and were audio tape-recorded. The FGDs were conducted at a research centre near participants' workplaces. They lasted approximately 60 minutes and were audio-recorded. A brief orientation of oral-fluid based HIVST was presented during FGDs but participants were not offered the test kits. During the FGDs, notes were taken by an experienced recorder and expanded immediately after the FGDs. The first author [BN] and two-trained research assistants (1 male, 1 female) conducted the FGDs and IDIs in Kiswahili.

Participants were allowed to respond spontaneously to each question and were not required to seek permission to speak or speak in a designated order. The facilitator encouraged all women to participate in the discussion by using probers and made efforts to provoke deviating perceptions.

Before the actual data collection, the data collection tools were pilot tested to check for clarity and internal consistency. After the pilot, a few corrections on the wordings were made on the data collection tools. Eight participants (4 males, 4 females) meeting the same eligibility criteria, as the main study participants were involved, which informed minor word

5.4 Data management and synthesis

We used the Framework Method for data management and synthesis. The Framework Method is a systematic and flexible approach and appropriate for analysing qualitative data. The Framework Method identifies commonalities and differences in qualitative data, focusing on relationships between different parts of the data. The Framework Method is divided into seven (7) phases, which provide the procedure for qualitative data analysis. The seven steps include (a) transcription, (b) familiarization of information, (c) coding, (d) developing the analytical framework, (e) applying the analytical framework, (f) charting data into framework matrix and (g) interpretation of data.

The purpose of using the framework approach is to draw descriptive and/or explanatory conclusions clustered around themes, to address the research question and the study aim by producing credible and relevant findings (Gale et al., 2013). In this study, the application of the framework method was as follows. In the first step, an independent translator translated the transcripts from Swahili into English. In the second step, two investigators independently examined the transcripts to ensure comparable formatting, until they were satisfied that any inconsistencies in formatting had been resolved. All transcripts were checked for errors by listening back to the audio-recordings and reading the transcripts simultaneously. In the third step, two investigators thoroughly read and re-read each transcript to become familiar with the whole data set. In the fourth step, two investigators coded three translated transcripts and an independent qualitative analyst verified the coded data. Discrepancies in coding were discussed among the three investigators and resolved through consensus. All three investigators agreed on a set of codes, each with a brief definition, which formed the initial analytical framework. In the fifth step, two investigators independently coded three more transcripts using the initial framework, taking care to note any new codes or impressions, which did not fit the existing set. The texts and the codes were read repeatedly to identify pre-defined themes based on the IBM theoretical model and emergent themes from the data. Thereafter, the three authors met to revise the initial framework to incorporate new and refined codes. The process of data refining, applying and refining the analytical framework was repeated until no new codes were generated. The final framework consisted of pre-defined themes and codes (Table 5.1). No emergent themes were identified from the data. This process allowed us to generate an interpretive code list, which we used to code all of the remaining transcripts. We attempted to maximize validity by translating the English version interview guides in Swahili, back translating into English and piloting testing in Swahili before data collection. Furthermore, notes were taken and expanded and the data collection process was recorded and applied consistent coding of the data to minimize the chance of getting invalid data. In-depth interviews and FGDs were analysed separately, because the unit of analysis was different. The analyses were brought together at the write-up phase

Table 5.1. Summary of pre-defined themes and codes from FGDs	
Pre-defined themes	**Codes**
Attitude about HIVST	
Experiential attitude	The emotional response related to the uptake of HIVST including enjoying the freedom to test oneself, relief to avoid needle pricks and fear of seeing blood.
Instrumental attitude	Attitude towards HIVST, with anticipated positive consequences, including self-testing at a place of one's choice, privacy and convenience, avoiding long queues; reducing time visiting health facilities; less testing and waiting time for test results; reducing counsellor's workload; reducing indirect costs.
Perceived norms towards HIVST	
Injunctive norms	A belief that significant people in their social environment, such as parents and peers, would approve (or disapprove) the use of HIVST.
Descriptive norms	An individual's belief about whether significant people in their social environment, such as parents and peers would use (or not use) HIVST.
Personal agency towards HIVST	
Perceived control	**Control belief:** A perceived likelihood that HIVST will empower people to self-test for HIV. HIVST is likely to minimize stigma; lack of counselling is likely to motivate people to use HIVST.
	Beliefs about the facilitators for performance: Easy access of kits; availability of self-test kits; disclosure of negative results; positive results triggers action; appropriate locations for delivery of HIVST; strategies for advocacy HIVST; strategies for linkage to HIV care.
	Beliefs about barriers to performance: Unaffordable kit price; poverty; illiteracy; poor eye-sight; cost-benefit of HIVST; lack of HIVST policy; lack of counselling & linkage to HIV care; limitations of rapid HIV tests.
Self-efficacy	The availability of face-to-face counselling will clear doubts about an individual's capacity to perform HIVST; correct information would increase HIVST knowledge and the capacity to perform HIVST; less confidence to use HIVST correctly when alone.

5.5 Ethical considerations

The study received ethical approval from the Kilimanjaro Christian Medical University College Research and Ethical Reviews Committee (CREC: 884; dated: 6/1/2016), National Institute of Medical Research, Tanzania (NIMRlHQIR.8a/Vol. IX/2454; dated: 18/4/2017) and University of Cape Town, South Africa (HREC REF: 737; dated: 9/11/2016). All respondents were informed of the study objectives, confidentiality and procedures for written informed consent. At the end of the FGDs and IDIs, participants received reimbursement of Tanzanian Shillings (TZS) 3,000/= (US$ 1= 2,000 TZS) for transport fare. To uphold anonymity, all FGD and IDI participants were given code numbers, which were used during

5.6 Results

Fifty-five (n=55) participants (FBWs= 16; MCPs=21; Key informants =18) were involved in the study, reflecting representation among participants across sex, age, education level, marital status and previous history of HIV testing. Five FBWs who were invited to attend did not participate because of lack of time on the day scheduled for FGDs. Among FBW's, 7 had primary education, 14 were unmarried and 10 had previously been tested or HIV. The mean age was 26 years. All MCPs who were invited to attend participated. Among MCPs, 10 had primary education, 12 were married and 12 had previously been tested for HIV. The mean age was 31 years. Among KIs, 12 were males, 17 had secondary education, 15 were married and 13 were employed with regular salary. The mean age of KIs was 52 years (Table 5.2).

Table 5.2. Characteristics of participants (n=55)

	Female Bar workers n (%)	Mountain climbing porters n (%)	Key informants n (%)
Sex			
Male	0(0.0)	21(100.0)	12(66.7)
Female	16(100.0)	0(0.0)	6(33.3)
Data collection methods			
In-depth interviews (IDIs)	0(0.0)	0(0.0)	18(100.0)
Focus group discussions (FGDs)	16(100.0)	21(100.0)	0(0.0)
Age			
Mean age in years (range)	26 years (18-34)	31 years (22-48)	52 years (29-77)
Education level			
Primary education	7(43.7)	10(47.6)	1(5.6)
Secondary education or higher	9(56.3)	11(52.4)	17(94.4)
Marital status			
Married	2(12.5)	12(57.1)	15(83.3)
Employment status			
Employed with a regular salary	16(100.0)	0(0.0)	13(72.2)
History of HIV testing			
Ever tested for HIV	10(62.5)	12(57.1)	N/A*

* Key informants were not asked about their previous history of HIV testing

KIs included one (1) HIV expert at the national level, three (3) HIV experts at the regional level, three (3) HIV experts at the district level, one (1) VCT counsellors, two (2) clinicians (1 in a public facility; 1 in a private facility), four (4) influential leaders (1= Imam; 1= HIV NGO representative; 1= local leader; and 1= chairperson of community advisory board), three (3) tourist experts and one (1) bar worker. All KIs who were invited to attend the interviews participated.

5.6.1 Attitude about HIVST

According to the IBM model, attitude towards a behaviour refers to experiential attitude (emotional response to the idea of engaging in a behaviour) and instrumental attitude

Male participants' emotional responses related to the uptake of HIVST included enjoying the freedom to test themselves after deciding to test for HIV. This was well illustrated in the following quote from a male participant: *"I would prefer self-testing because I will have the freedom to test myself, once I have decided to test for HIV"* (30-year-old man, FGD).

Most female participants expressed anticipated relief to avoid needle pricks by using an oral-fluid self-test and fear of seeing blood. This observation was well described by a female participant who said: "By *using this [oral-HIVST]... you do not need to prick yourself to get a blood sample but you collect a sample from the mouth to test for HIV. I will prefer it [oral-HIVST] because I dislike seeing blood and I also fear needle pricks*" (34-year-old woman, FGD).

Female participants expressed that their ability to self- test for HIV would increase their trust and acceptability of their test results:

> *"First, I will have the ability to test myself. Secondly, I will trust my HIV self-test results because I am the one who has done the test, which is different from if someone would have taken my blood or a sample from the mouth and go to test for HIV. So if I test myself whatever the test result may be I will accept it"* (23-year-old woman, FGD).

Other positive consequences of HIVST that were anticipated by both female and male participants included privacy during testing, avoidance of long queues, reduced time spent travelling to and from health facilities, reduced time spent waiting for test results, a reduced counsellor's workload and reduced indirect costs related to transporting to facilities. Male participants particularly valued the privacy and convenience that they anticipated was a consequence of being able to test them:

"First, I will test in the privacy of my house and this [HIVST] will reduce the costs of transport of going to the health facility to test for HIV. Secondly, I will avoid the long queues in the health facilities, while waiting for testing services. Thirdly, it will reduce the time I would use to go to the health facility and also I will use less time to test and get my results" (48-year-old man, FGD).

Anticipated positive consequences particularly valued by female participants were reduced transport costs to visit a testing point. This was well explained by a middle-aged female participant who said: *"If I buy this kit [self-test] and test myself at home, I will reduce the cost of transport to go to test at a health facility or stand-alone clinic"* (30-year-old

Additionally, a key informant observed that HIVST might free counsellors' time previously spent on testing HIV-negative individuals and hence reduce their workload:"[...] *from our side [counsellors] we will have fewer clients to attend, which will reduce the workload*"(52-year-old counsellor, IDI).

5.6.2 Perceived norms about HIVST

It is theorized that injunctive norms (beliefs about what significant others think one should do regarding a behaviour) and descriptive norms (individual's perception about the extent to which significant others will perform the recommended behaviour) about HIVST will influence the intention to perform HIVST. Participants expressed perceived norms that were supportive of HIVST. None mentioned norms that were not supportive of HIVST.

Injunctive norms

Participants expressed a belief that people in their social environment, such as parents and peers, would approve their uptake of HIVST. The belief supportive of HIVST was well illustrated in the following quote: *"I know my mother would approve that I use HIVST to test for HIV. She always insists that I should be careful with my health because we work in a very risky environment for HIV infection"* (25-year-old woman, FGD).

Subjective norms

Some female respondents expressed the belief that significant people such as relatives or friends would accept and take up HIVST. This positive belief was illustrated in the following quote: *"I think relatives or friends will see it [HIVST] as an additional approach that may increase testing options, which is easy to use and needs less time to know their HIV status"* (24-year-old woman, FGD).

5.6.3 Personal agency toward HIVST

Control belief

Male participants agreed that testing for HIV on their own would facilitate the uptake of HIVST. Men felt that taking control of their testing and making positive choices derived from using the HIVST kits was a positive feature of HIVST and a first step to know one's HIV status:

> *"HIVST is very important to me because it will empower me to test for HIV whenever I decide to test. This could be like the first step to know my HIV status before I decide to go to test for HIV at a health facility or testing centres"* (21-year-old man, FGD).

Some KIs perceived that the introduction of HIVST would likely minimize the stigma associated with HIV testing and this would facilitate uptake: "*I think HIVST will reduce stigma in the community because my results will remain my secret I am sure no one will*

Interestingly, a KI observed that young people might be motivated to use HIVST because of the lack of counselling since they have no time to wait: *"Some people may be motivated to use HIVST because of lack of counselling, particularly young people who have no time to wait"* (54 -year-old man, IDI).

Some KIs believed that monetary incentives and the availability of social support for those who test HIV positive would facilitate acceptance of HIV testing. A male informant said: "[...] *for example provide incentives [monetary] for those who will agree to test for HIV. Also, there should be social support for those who will be HIV positive, such as diet, financial assistance and counselling*"(40-year-old man, IDI).

Conversely, a male KI mentioned monetary incentives as a potential impediment:

> *"Initially, incentives may work to motivate people to use HIVST kits to know their HIV status. However, this may not be sustainable in the long run, if you consider the issue of ART adherence for example. What I believe is that clients should know that HIV testing is beneficial to their overall health status and they would proactively seek care and treatment*"(58 -year-old man, IDI).

Beliefs about the facilitators for performance

Some KIs believed that the features of oral-fluid HIV self-testing that would facilitate uptake were that it would be easy to use, painless and less invasive compared with finger pricks for blood-based testing. A male KI however perceived that the stated preference of oral-fluid test might hinder HIVST uptake because of concerns around accuracy:

> "*My concern here will be the accuracy of the results from these two samples. I am not sure if the results will be the same or different. However, from our clients' perspectives, I think most will believe the results from the blood compared with the results from a sample from the mouth (oral-fluid sample). The reason is simple-the the current rapid test that we are using we collect a blood sample for testing, so clients are used to that. Another reason is their understanding that the viruses are in the blood and not in the oral-fluids! If we introduce taking a sample from the mouth (oral-fluid sample) to test for HIV, it will take time and effort to convince clients that it is possible to test HIV from a sample taken from the mouth*"(58-year-old man, IDI).

Female participants mentioned that features of an HIVST distribution strategy that would facilitate uptake were the availability of accessible locations for distribution, interventions to advocate for HIVST, making people aware of HIVST and interventions to ensure and linkage from HIVST to HIV prevention treatment and care

Female participants believed that easy access of HIVST kits and disclosure of a negative HIV test result has a positive effect in performing HIVST: "*I do not think at the hospital it will be easy. I think at the drug shop or pharmacy is much easier because I will go there at any time and buy my kit and go back home to test*" (29-year-old woman, FGD).

Another female participant observed: *"[...]once you test and find that you are HIV negative, then you disclose your test results to your male partner and he would be motivated to do self-testing"* (30-year-old woman, FGD).

Female participants perceived the results of the self-test might facilitate linkage to care. A female discussant stated: *"If I find that I am HIV positive, I will go to the health facility to confirm my test results"* (32-year-old, woman, FGD).

Also, female participants commonly cited pharmacies, or drug shops and workplaces as appropriate locations for distribution of HIVST that might facilitate the uptake of HIVST. A young woman explained: *"I think the appropriate place should be in pharmacies or drug shops or chemists etc*." (25-year-old woman, FGD).

Some KIs perceived that the availability of appropriate locations for and strategies of distribution of HIVST kits would facilitate uptake of HIVST and that these included community-based distributors, integration into existing services and outreach community-based interventions and vending machines and kiosks.
A male KI elaborated: "*For HIV self-test to retain its true meaning, services must be available close to residential areas [...], so delivery could be door-to-door. We have the home-based care service (HBC) and the home-based care attendants can move from house to house to supply the self-test kits*" (38-year-old man, IDI).

Conversely, another KI perceived that public distribution of HIVST kits may negatively impact the uptake of HIVST:

> *"What is important I think is how the HIVST kits will be distributed. If the HIVST kits will be distributed in public places where there is a possibility of other people seeing the collection of the kits, no one will be willing to come forward to collect the kits"*(58-year-old clinician, IDI).

KIs perceived that strategies for advocacy and raising awareness of HIVST, including the use of influential leaders, use of existing peer networks and effective communication, might positively affect HIVST uptake KIs cited the role of influential leaders in raising awareness

A woman informant explained:

> *'The community leaders should be the first group of people to be trained on HIVST in the community. The community leaders would include priests, pastors, sheikhs, politicians and the so-called: 'influential people' –people who are respected in the community. Once they* [influential leaders] *are aware of the HIVST they will play a very important role in creating awareness in the community because they have many followers who trust them* [influential leaders]" (62-year-old woman, IDI).

Finally, KIs mentioned a variety of strategies that may facilitate linkage to HIV prevention, treatment and care following HIVST. The strategies were well described by a female key informant in the following quote:

"[...]if we involve community health workers in the distribution of the HIVST test kits, then it will be easy for the same community health workers to follow-up clients who have requested for the test kits and ask them if they have tested and if they have sought care. Another alternative could be to ask clients to return the self-test kits to the pharmacy or drug shop after a certain period, for example, 3 days and recorded in a register. Another alternative could be the use of mobile applications or services such as phone calls or text messages to monitor clients and link them to HIV prevention, care and treatment services" (50-year-old woman, IDI).

Beliefs about barriers to performance

A common impediment to the uptake of HIVST cited by most female participants was the cost of buying the self-test kits. A young woman explained: "[...] *most people in the rural settings are poor. Therefore, if these [self-testing kits] will be sold in pharmacies, it may be difficult for most people to afford"* (23-year old woman, FGD).

Most KIs suggested no-cost or very low cost kits should be provided through government subsidies or health schemes to circumvent the cost of buying the self-test kits. A male informant explained: *"I think health insurance schemes could cover for the cost of buying the HIVST kits. For example, most porters are covered by a health insurance scheme called: Micro Health Initiative, which pays for their treatment when they fall sick"* (44-year-old man, IDI).

Another impediment to the uptake of HIVST, mentioned by some female participants, was the cost-benefit of buying self-test kits or food. A women participant said: *'I don't want a*

Participants mentioned other constraints that may hinder the uptake of HIVST including: illiteracy, physical disabilities such as poor eyesight and fear of HIV positive results. A young man explained: '*Most people, particularly in the rural areas are illiterate; they cannot read a newspaper. How could they be able to read and follow the instructions of how to perform self-testing?*'(24-year-old man, FGD).

Another male participant added: '[...] *the problem will be to people, who have eyesight problems, then it will be difficult for them to perform HIVST and they may need assistance*' (22-year-old man, FGD).

A male KI cited fear of HIV positive results:

> '*Fear of HIV positive results is what makes most people not to test for HIV. The main reason for this fear is anticipated-stigma-whereby people think that if they are diagnosed HIV positive, other people will know and isolate them either at the workplaces or in their community*' (52-year-old man, IDI).

KIs perceived lack of policy on HIVST might hinder uptake. A male HIV expert had this to say: '[...] *lack of policy on HIVST may be a barrier to self-testing*' (50-year-old man, IDI).

Male participants raised concerns regarding the quality of HIVST kits because of a lack of regulatory mechanisms and past experiences of buying fake drugs: '*We have experiences of buying fake drugs from some drug shops / or pharmacies. What will prevent them not to sell fake self-testing kits?*' (31-year-old man, FGD).

A KI perceived lack of counselling and linkage to care as another constraint to the uptake of HIVST, leading to missing or delayed initiation to treatment: '[...], *I anticipate lack of linkage to care, particularly for those who will test HIV positive, if there will be no follow-up mechanisms. This may lead to missing or delayed initiation of treatment*' (52-year-old woman HIV expert, IDI).

A female KI expressed her concern related to the limitations of HIVST as a screening test and a follow-up visit to a health facility for a confirmatory test in case of a reactive result:

"*My concern is the fact that HIV self-testing is a screening procedure. If my test result is reactive, then I need to go to the health facility again for a confirmatory test. My other concern is that HIVST tests like any other rapid HIV tests have a limitation of not detecting*

Self-efficacy towards HIVST

Male participants were confident in their capacity to use the HIVST kits. Some male participants stated their preference for face-to-face counselling with a trained counsellor to clear doubts about an individual's performance with HIVST kits.

A male participant explained: *"Wherever the self-test kits would be available, clients must receive counselling and a demonstration on how to use the self-test kits before they buy the kits and test for HIV. Once clients receive all the necessary information, self-testing correctly for HIV is possible"* (24-year-old man, FGD).

However, some female participants were less confident in their capacity to use the HIVST kits correctly when alone. Their lack of confidence in their capacity to use the kits may lead to potential mistakes, which would reduce their trust in the self-test results:

"I will not be confident to test myself as if I will go to ANGAZA (a stand-alone VCT site)...that the instrument [HIVST] has shown correctly the results...maybe I have made a certain mistake or there may be something which I have done wrong..." (28-year-old woman, FGD).

5.7 Discussion

This formative study aimed to explore KIs knowledge about the motivation and beliefs of the community on HIVST and FBWs and MCPs attitudes, perceived norms and personal agency beliefs related to HIVST uptake in northern Tanzania.

Despite the lack of HIVST awareness in Tanzania, most participants expressed positive experiential and instrumental attitudes towards HIVST. Positive attitudes towards HIVST were primarily related to enjoying the freedom to test for HIV in privacy and at a convenient place of their choice, and relief to avoid needle pricks by using the oral-fluid sample, which is a less invasive and painless procedure. These findings are in line with studies done in other settings (Choko et al., 2011, Pe´rez et al., 2016, Conserve et al., 2018).

In this study, health care providers viewed HIVST as an opportunity to ease their workload giving them time to deal with individuals with HIV-positive results. In most LMICs such as Tanzania, there is a shortage of health care providers including counsellors, who are face heavy-workloads in clinical settings leading to burnout syndrome and resulting in inefficiency (Maestad et al., 2010). Therefore, HIVST will enable counsellors to have more time focusing on those with reactive results in need of confirmatory testing and initiation of ART (WHO 2016).

Most participants expressed beliefs about the facilitators for the uptake of HIVST. Some of the facilitators for the uptake of HIVST are more salient for men since evidence suggests that time-consuming activities, for example, discourage men from seeking HIV testing services (Indravudh et al., 2017). Several studies have documented men's reluctance to go to test at an HIV testing point. Men's reluctance is because of the so-called 'masculinity'-which is a social construct around male ego of not showing their feelings in public and the perception that HIV testing is a woman's domain (Grabbe et al., 2010, Njau et al., 2012, Morfaw et al., 2013, Matovu et al., 2015, Choko et al., 2017).

Findings from this study highlight that HIVST is likely to minimize the stigma associated with HIV testing at a testing point or facility by reducing visibility associated with visiting clinical settings, lack of confidentiality of test results and long waiting times. This observation corroborates previous studies on stigma related to accessing HTS in clinical settings (Njau et al., 2012, Mukolo et al., 2013, Musheke et al., 2013, Ostermann et al., 2014).

Young people perceived a lack of counselling favorable because they usually do not have time to wait long at HIV testing points. This observation is in line with findings from other settings, whereby people dislike face-to-face counselling because it is repetitive, frustrating, intrusive and time-consuming (Indravudh et al., 2017).

Besides, the different perceptions on preferences between oral-fluid specimens compared with finger prick reported in this study must be addressed to correct misconceptions related to the accuracy of HIVST test results and different specimen collection methods (Mukolo et al., 2013, Njau et al., 2014, Ostermann et al., 2014).

Since HIVST is not familiar in Tanzania, and to facilitate advocacy and awareness creation of HIVST to increase uptake of HIV testing, a peer-based approach for HIVST education and promotion could improve target population behaviours towards HIV testing. Existing evidence suggests that the use of peer-educators for the promotion of health behaviour-related interventions are highly effective in behaviour change, such as HIV testing (Ford et al., 2008, Geibel et al., 2012, Onyango et al., 2016, Chanda et al., 2017, Oldenburg et al., 2017).

Different service delivery approaches for HIVST were cited by most participants as potential facilitators for effective linkage to HIV prevention, care and treatment. For example, using of door-to-door distribution of HIVST by trained community-based distributors was viewed as an effective strategy of linkage to care, by offering a proactive follow-up, including post-test counselling and assistance on referrals for a confirmatory test (WHO 2016)

Furthermore, the use of mobile applications such as phone calls or short messages services (SMS) is also recommended to facilitate linkage to HIV prevention, care and treatment. Other studies have documented the use of mobile applications as a cost-effective intervention in increasing HIV testing (de Tolly et al., 2012, Kelvin et al., 2017).

Participants in the current study also reported commonly cited constraints that may hinder HIVST uptake across the literature. Examples include high cost of buying self-test kits, and limitations of self-test kits, in not detecting acute HIV infections. Other constraints were missing or delaying treatment among HIV-positive individuals that may arise following self-testing due to lack of pre and post-test counselling and strategies for linkage to care (Musheke et al., 2013, Pai et al., 2013, WHO 2016). To circumvent constraints such as the cost of buying self-test kits, implementation of low or no cost HIVST kits, through subsidies or insurance mechanisms to cover for the cost of buying the kits may be an alternative approach (Musheke et al., 2013, Pai et al., 2013, Choko et al., 2017).

Our results showed mixed findings on the participants' confidence in their capacity to use the HIVST. Interestingly, men compared to women, reported high confidence in using HIVST correctly after face-to-face counselling with a trained counsellor, parallel to findings from other settings (Pai, et al., 2013, Choko et al., 2017). Evidence suggests that lack of instructions-for-use and/ or lack of demonstration on how to perform and interpret the self-test results contribute to user errors (Pai et al., 2013). To address the low confidence in using HIVST correctly, particularly among women, interventionists must consider providing additional guidance to potential self-testers on how to perform the HIVST (Pai et al., 2013, Choko et al., 2017).

Limitations

The current study has limitations worth noting. The findings might be affected by selection bias because we sought to include a purposive sample of study participants, but other potentially relevant participants with different views on the study topic may not have been adequately represented in the sample. It is important to remember the limits of focus group data. While focus groups are very good at uncovering the range of experience, they are not good at uncovering how common any one experience might be. This is because not every person was asked or required to answer every question. A participant's silence does not necessarily mean that they did not have an opinion or an experience.

In addition, we did not assess the participant's knowledge about HIVST, the ability to use and follow HIVST instructions or interpret HIVST results. Future studies should explore target population's perceptions towards HIVST after viewing different demonstration materials (e.g. videos, print materials, simulation on how to use self-test kits) to determine which methods

Finally, because of the sensitive nature of the topic under study, there was a possibility of participants' giving answers to satisfy the facilitator.

5.8 Conclusions

The findings from this study suggest that a BCI based on IBM to increase HIVST uptake may be acceptable in this study setting. The majority of participants reported positive attitudes, supportive perceived norms and self-efficacy towards HIVST uptake. The study findings were considered in the designing and development of the BCI described in details in **Chapter Six**.

References

Abamecha, F., A. Godesso and E. Girma (2013). "Intention to voluntary HIV counselling and testing(VCT) among health professionals in Jimma zone, Ethiopia: the Theory of Planned Behaviour (TPB) perspective." BMC Public Health **13**(140): 1-7.

Administration(FDA)., U. F. a. D. (2012). OraQuick In-Home HIV test summary of safety and effectiveness. Silver Spring: FDA; 2012.

Ao, T. T., N. E. Sam, E. J. Masenga, G. R. Seage and S. H. Kapiga (2006). "Human Immunodeficiency Virus Type 1 Among Bar and Hotel Workers in Northern Tanzania: The Role of Alcohol, Sexual Behavior and Herpes Simplex Virus Type 2." Sexually Transmitted Diseases **33**(3): 163-169.

Bandura, A. (2004). "Health promotion by social cognitive means." Health Educ Behav **31**(2): 143-164.

Baranowski, T., C. Perry and G. Parcel (2002). How individuals, environments and health behavior interact: Social Cognitive Theory. In K. Glanz, B. Rimer & F. M. Lewis(Eds.), Health Behavior and Health Education: Theory, research and practice (3rded., pp. 165-184). San Francisco: Jossey-Bass.

Chanda, M. M., K. F. Ortblad, M. Mwale, S. Chongo, C. Kanchele, N. Kamungoma, et al. (2017). "HIV self-testing among female sex workers in Zambia: A cluster randomized controlled trial." PLoS Medicine **14**(11): e1002442.

Choko, A. T., N. Desmond, E. L. Webb, K. Chavula, S. Napierala-Mavedzenge, C. A. Gaydos, et al. (2011). "The Uptake and Accuracy of Oral Kits for HIV Self-Testing in High HIV Prevalence Setting: A Cross-Sectional Feasibility Study in Blantyre, Malawi." PLoS Medicine **8**(10).

Choko, A. T., M. K. Kumwenda, C. C. Johnson, D. W. Sakala, M. C. Chikalipo, K. Fielding, et al. (2017). "Acceptability of woman-delivered HIV self-testing to the male partner and additional interventions: a qualitative study of antenatal care participants in Malawi." Journal of the International Aids Society **20**(1): 1-10.

Conserve, D., L. Kajula, T. Yamanis and S. Maman (2016). "Formative Research to Develop Human Immunodeficiency Virus (HIV) Self-Testing Intervention Among Networks of Men in Dar es Salaam, Tanzania: A Mixed Methods Approach." Open Forum Infectious Diseases, Volume 3, Issue suppl_1, **3**,(1,): 518.

Conserve, D. F., D. Alemu, T. Yamanis, S. Maman and L. Kajula (2018). "He Told Me to Check My Health": A Qualitative Exploration of Social Network Influence on Men's HIV Testing Behavior and HIV Self-Testing Willingness in Tanzania." American Journal of Men's Health.

Conserve, D. F., K. E. Muessig, L. L. Maboko, S. Shirima, M. N. Kilonzo, S. Maman, et al. (2018). "Mate Yako Afya Yako: Formative research to develop the Tanzania HIV self-testing education and promotion (Tanzania STEP) project for men." PLoS ONE.

Creswell, J. W. and D. L. Miller (2000). "Determining validity in qualitative inquiry." Theory Into Practice **39**(3): 124-130.

de Tolly, K., D. Skinner, V. Nembaware and P. Benjamin (2012). "Investigation into the use of short message services to expand uptake of human immunodeficiency virus testing and whether content and dosage have an impact." Telemed Journal of Education of Health **18**(1): 18-23.

Fishbein, M. (2007). A Reasoned Action Approach: Some Issues, Questions and Clarifications. Prediction and Change of Health Behaviour: Applying the Reasoned Action Approach. I. Ajzen, D. Albaraccin and R.Hornik., Hillsdale, N.J.: Erlbaum,2007.

Fishbein M and I Azjen (1975) Belief Attitude Intention and Behaviour: An Introduction to

Fishbein, M. and J. N. Cappella (2006). "The role of theory in developing effective health communications." Journal of Communication **56**(S1-S17.): S1-S17.
Ford, K., D. N. Wirawan, W. Suastina, B. D. Reed and P. Muliawan (2008). "Evaluation of a peer education programme for female sex workers in Bali, Indonesia. ." International Journal of STD AIDS **11**: 731–733.
Gale, N. K., G. Heath, E. Cameron, S. Rashid and S. Redwood (2013). "Using the framework method for the analysis of qualitative data in multi-disciplinary health research." BMC Medical Research Methodology **13:**(117).
Geibel, S., N. King'ola, M. Temmerman and S. Luchters (2012). "The impact of peer outreach on HIV knowledge and prevention behaviours of male sex workers in Mombasa, Kenya. ." Sexually Transmitted Infections **88**: 357–362.
Glanz, K., B. K. Rimer and K. Viswanath (2008). Health behavior and health education: theory, research and practice. San Francisco, Jossey-Bass.
Godin, G. and G. Kok (1996). "The theory of planned behaviour: a review of applications to health-related behaviours." American Journal of Health Promotion. **11**: 87-98.
Grabbe, K. L., N. Menzies, M. Taegtmeyer, G. Emukule, P. Angala, I. Mwega, et al. (2010). "Increasing access to HIV counselling and testing through mobile services in Kenya: strategies, utilization and cost-effectiveness." Journal of Acquired Immune Deficiency Syndromes **54**(3): 317-323.
Indravudh, P. P., E. L. Sibanda, M. d'Elbee, M. K. Kumwenda, B. Ringwald, G. Maringwa, et al. (2017). "'I will choose when to test, where I want to test': investigating young people's preferences for HIV self-testing in Malawi and Zimbabwe." AIDS **31 Suppl 3**: S203-S212.
Jennings, L., D. F. Conserve, J. Merrill, L. Kajula, J. Iwelunmor, S. Linnemayr, et al. (2017). "Perceived Cost Advantages and Disadvantages of Purchasing HIV Self- Testing Kits among Urban Tanzanian Men: An Inductive Content Analysis." Journal of AIDS & Clinical Research **08**(08).
Johnson, C., R. Baggaley, S. Forsythe, H. van Rooyen, N. Ford, S. Napierala Mavedzenge, et al. (2014). "Realizing the Potential for HIV Self-Testing." AIDS Behavior.
Johnson, C. C., C. Kennedy, V. A. Fonner, N. Siegfried, C. Figueroa, S. Dalal, et al. (2017). "Examining the effects of HIV self-testing compared to standard HIV testing services: a systematic review and meta-analysis." Journal of the International Aids Society **20**(1).
Kakoko, C., A. Astrom, L. Lugoe and T. Lie (2006). "Predicting intended use of Voluntary counselling and testing services in Tanzanian teachers using the theory of planned behaviour." Social Science & Medicine **63(4)**:: 991-999.
Kapiga, S. H., N. E. Sam, J. F. Shao, B. Renjifo, E. J. Massenga, I. E. Kiwelu, et al. (2002). "HIV-1 Epidemic Among Female Bar Workers and Hotel Workers in Northern Tanzania: Risk Factors and Opportunities for Prevention." Journal of Acquired Immune Deficiency Syndromes **29(4)**: 409-417.
Kelvin, E. A., G. George, E. Mwai, E. N. Nyaga, J. E. Mantell, M. L. Romo, et al. (2017). "Offering Self-administered Oral HIV Testing as a Choice to Truck Drivers in Kenya: Predictors of Uptake and Need for Guidance While Self-testing." AIDS Behavior.
Kumwenda, M., A. Munthali, M. Phiri, D. Mwale, T. Gutteberg, E. MacPherson, et al. (2014). "Factors shaping initial decision-making to self-test amongst cohabiting couples in urban Blantyre, Malawi." AIDS Behavior **18 Suppl 4**: S396-404.
Lyamuya, J. E., B. Njau, D. J. Damian and T. Mtuy (2017). "Sociodemographic and Other Characteristics Associated With Behavioural Risk Factors of HIV Infection Among Male Mountain-Climbing Porters in Kilimanjaro Region, Tanzania." East African Health Research Journal: 1-8.
Maestad, O., G. Torsvik and A. Aakvik (2010). "Overworked? On the relationship between workload and health care performance." Journal of Health Economy **29**(5): 686-698.
Maheswaran, H., S. Petrou, P. MacPherson, A. T. Choko, F. Kumwenda, D. G. Lalloo, et al. (2016). "Cost and quality of life analysis of HIV self-testing and facility-based HIV testing and counselling in Blantyre, Malawi." BMC Medicine **14**: 34.
Matovu, J. K. B., J. Todd, R. K. Wanyenze, F. Wabwire-Mangen and D. Serwadda (2015). "Correlates of previous couples' HIV counselling and testing uptake among married individuals in three HIV prevalence strata in Rakai, Uganda." Glob Health Action **8**.
Mirkuzie, A. H., M. M. Sisay, K. M. Moland and A. N. Astrom (2011). "Applying the theory of planned behaviour to explain HIV testing in antenatal settings in Addis Ababa - a cohort study." BMC Health Services Research **11**(196).
Morfaw, F., L. Mbuagbaw, L. Thabane, C. Rodrigues, A. P. Wunderlich, P. Nana, et al. (2013). "Male involvement in prevention programs of mother to child transmission of HIV: a systematic review to identify barriers and facilitators." Syst Rev **2**: 5.
Mukolo, A., M. Blevins, B. Victor, H. N. Paulin, L. M. Vaz, M. Sidat, et al. (2013). "Community stigma endorsement and voluntary counselling and testing behavior and attitudes among female heads of household in Zambezia Province, Mozambique." BMC Public Health **13**: 1155.
Mukolo, A., I. Torres, R. M. Bechtel, M. Sidat and A. E. Vergara (2013). "Consensus on context-specific strategies for reducing the stigma of human immunodeficiency virus/acquired

Murray, A., L. Toledo, E. E. Brown and M. Y. Sutton (2017). "We as Black Men Have to Encourage Each other:" Facilitators and barriers associated with HIV testing among Black/African American men in rural Florida." Journal of Health Care for the Poor and Underserved **28**(1): 487– 498.
Musheke, M., H. Ntalasha, S. Gari, O. McKenzie, V. Bond, A. Martin-Hilber, et al. (2013). "A systematic review of qualitative findings on factors enabling and deterring uptake of HIV testing in Sub-Saharan Africa." BMC Public Health **13**: 220.
Njau, B., J. Ostermann, D. Brown, A. Muhlbacher, E. Reddy and N. Thielman (2014). "HIV testing preferences in Tanzania: a qualitative exploration of the importance of confidentiality, accessibility and quality of service." BMC Public Health **14**: 838.
Njau, B., M. H. Watt, J. Ostermann, R. Manongi and K. J. Sikkema (2012). "Perceived acceptability of home-based couples voluntary HIV counselling and testing in Northern Tanzania." AIDS Care **24**(4): 413-419.
Oldenburg, C. E., K. F. Ortblad, M. M. Chanda, K. Mwanda, W. Nicodemus, R. Sikaundi, et al. (2017). "Zambian Peer Educators for HIV Self-Testing (ZEST) study rationale and design of a cluster-randomized trial of HIV self-testing among female sex workers in Zambia." BMJ Open **7**(4): e014780.
Onyango, M. A., Y. Adu-Sarkodie, T. Agyarko-Poku, M. K. Asafo, J. Sylvester, P. Wondergem, et al. (2016). "It's all about making a life": poverty, HIV, violence and other vulnerabilities faced by young female sex workers in Kumasi, Ghana. ." Journal of AIDS **68**: S131–137.
Ostermann J, Whetten K, Reddy E, Pence B, Weinhold A, Itemba D, et al. (2014). "Treatment retention and care transitions during and after the scale-up of HIV care and treatment in Northern Tanzania." AIDS Care. 2014;26(11):1352-8. Doi: 10.1080/09540121.2014.882493.
Ostermann, J., B. Njau, D. S. Brown, A. Muhlbacher and N. Thielman (2014). "Heterogeneous HIV testing preferences in an urban setting in Tanzania: results from a discrete choice experiment." PLoS ONE **9**(3): e92100.
Ostermann, J., B. Njau, T. Mtuy, D. S. Brown, A. Muhlbacher and N. Thielman (2015). "One size does not fit all: HIV testing preferences differ among high-risk groups in Northern Tanzania." AIDS Care **27**(5): 595-603.
Pai, N. P., J. Sharma, S. Shivkumar, S. Pillay, C. Vadnais, L. Joseph, et al. (2013). "Supervised and Unsupervised Self-Testing for HIV in High- and Low-Risk Populations: A Systematic Review." PLoS Medicine **10(4):** : e1001414. .
Pant Pai, N., T. Behlim, L. Abrahams, C. Vadnais, S. Shivkumar, S. Pillay, et al. (2013). "Will an Unsupervised Self-Testing Strategy for HIV Work in Health Care Workers of South Africa? A Cross-Sectional Pilot Feasibility Study." PLoS ONE **8**(11).
Pe´rez, G. M., V. Cox, T. Ellman, A. Moore, G. Patten and A. Shroufi, et al. (2016). "'I Know that I Do Have HIV but Nobody Saw Me': Oral HIV Self-Testing in an Informal Settlement in South Africa." PLoS ONE **11**(4): e0152653.
Peaty, D. (2010). "Kilimanjaro Tourism and What It Means for Local Porters and the Local Environment." Journal of Ritsumeikan Social Sciences and Humanities **4**: 1-12.
Singleton, R. A. and B. C. Straits (2005). Approaches to Social Research. New York, USA., Oxford University Press, Inc.
Siu, G. E., D. Wight and J. A. Seeley (2014). "Masculinity, social context and HIV testing: an ethnographic study of men in Busia district, rural eastern Uganda." BMC Public Health **14**(1): 33.
THIS (2017). TANZANIA HIV IMPACT SURVEY(THIS) 2016-2017: PRELIMINARY FINDINGS. Dar-es-Salaam, Tanzania, Ministry of Health, Community Development, Gender, Elderly and Children (MoHCDGEC) and the Ministry of Health (MoH) Zanzibar through the National Bureau of Statistics (NBS) and the Office of Chief Government Statistician (OCGS)**:** 1-6.
UNAIDS (2014). A short Technical Update on Self-Testing for HIV, the Joint United Nations Programme on HIV/AIDS World Health Organization.
UNAIDS (2015). HOW AIDS CHANGED EVERYTHING: MDG 6: 15 YEARS, 15 LESSONS OF HOPE FROM THE AIDS RESPONSE, JOINT UNAIDS & WHO, Geneva Switzerland.
UNAIDS (2017). "UNAIDS Data ".
UNAIDS/WHO (2010). Towards universal access-scaling up priority HIV/AIDS interventions in the health sector-progress report. Geneva, World Health Organization.
The United Republic of Tanzania and the Ministry of Health and Social Welfare National Aids Control Programme (2007). Guidelines on HIV Testing and Counselling in Clinical settings, Dar es Salaam, Tanzania.
United Republic of Tanzania National Bureau of Statistics and ICF (2013). HIV/AIDS Malaria Indicator Survey 2011-12. In Dar es Salaam, Tanzania: Tanzania Commission for AIDS, ZAC, NBS, OCGS and ICF International;2013.
The United Republic of Tanzania, N. B. S. (2012). 2012 Tanzania Population and Housing Census Dar es Salaam, National Bureau of Statistics.
Wanyenze, R. K., J. A. Hahn, C. A. Liechty, K. Ragland, A. Ronald, H. Mayanja-Kizza, et al. (2011) "Linkage to HIV care and survival following inpatient HIV counselling and testing " AIDS

World Health Organization (2016). Guidelines on HIV self-testing and partner notification: supplement to consolidated guidelines on HIV testing services. France., World Health Organization, Geneva 27, Switzerland.: 1-104.

Xun, H., D. Kang, T. Huang, Y. Qian, X. Li, E. C. Wilson, et al. (2013). "Factors Associated with the Willingness to Accept Oral Fluid HIV rapid Testing among Most-at-Risk Populations in China." PLoS ONE **8**(11): e80594.

Zanolini, A., J. Chipungu, M. J. Vinikoor, S. Bosomprah, M. Mafwenko, C. B. Holmes, et al. (2017). "HIV Self-Testing in Lusaka Province, Zambia: Acceptability, Comprehension of Testing Instructions and Individual Preferences for Self-Test Kit Distribution in a Population-Based Sample of Adolescents and Adults." AIDS Research and Human Retroviruses.

CHAPTER SIX

6.0 Developing a behaviour change intervention to increase HIVST uptake and linkage to HIV prevention, care and treatment among female bar workers and male mountain climbing porters in Northern Tanzania

Chapter Six describes how the behaviour change intervention (BCI) to increase HIVST uptake and linkage to HIV prevention, care and treatment among FBWs and MCPs in Northern Tanzania was designed based on the Integrated Behavior Model (IBM) and the formative research and synthesis of evidence on HIVST. The process of intervention development was guided by the PRECEDE-PROCEED planning model (Green and Kreuter 1999).

6.1 Introduction

Guidance for developing complex interventions such as those focusing on the uptake of HIV testing, advocate the use of behavioural change theories in the intervention development process (Godin et al., 2008, Hoffmann et al., 2014), because interventions are more likely to be effective if they target causal determinants of behaviour and behaviour change. Behavioural change theories are useful in gaining an understanding of the causal mechanisms (Godin et al., 2008).

Many intervention studies however, do not report an adequate description of justification, the development procedures and sufficient depiction of the intervention components, methods of delivery and the context in which it is implemented to support replication and/or modification of interventions (Hoffmann et al., 2014). Poor planning, lack of a link to behavioural theories and lack of formative research involving potential users may account for the gap (Godin et al., 2008).

Several theoretical approaches exist that could be used to inform the development of interventions. The purposes of using theoretical approaches in intervention development include (a) describe and/or guiding the process of translating evidence into practice, (b) understand and / or explaining what influences implementation outcomes and (c) evaluate implementation. To achieve the purpose of using theoretical approaches in intervention development, IBM was used. In brief, the IBM includes constructs from several behavioural change theories including the Theory of Reasoned Action (TRA), Theory of Planned Behavior (TPB), Health Belief Model (HBM) and Social Cognitive Theory

IBM, which is a useful framework to identify specific key beliefs on which to focus on intervention development, is also a strategy for behaviour change. Evidence suggests that the motivation or intention to engage in health-related behaviour is the strongest facilitator of behaviour change (Fishbein and Azjen 1975, Bandura 2004, Azjen 2006, Fishbein 2007). The IBM consists of three key constructs: attitude, social norms/influence and personal agency (detailed description in **Chapter One**). The aim of using the IBM in this study was to identify specific key beliefs underlying the IBM constructs that best explain the target population's level of motivation and focus for the BCI. To guide the process of developing and planning the BCI, this project followed the PRECEDE-PROCEED model (Glanz et al., 2008).

The PRECEDE-PROCEED model was used as a 'road map' and the main purpose was to provide a structure for applying the IBM construct systematically for guidance on the development of and process and outcome evaluation of the HIVST intervention.

6.2 Application of the PRECEDE-PROCEED model

6.2.1 Phase 1: Identifying the evidence-practice gap on HIVST uptake

In phase 1 of this project, the focus was to understand the existing social context related to current HIV testing practices and to identify and evaluate factors that may affect HIVST uptake and linkage to HIV prevention, care and treatment. To identify the evidence-practice gap in the existing social context related to the current HIV testing practices and factors that may affect HIVST uptake and linkage to HIV prevention, care and treatment, two activities were undertake (a) A systematic review to determine the effects of HIVST on the uptake of HIV testing and yield of new HIV positive diagnoses, social harms and linkage to antiretroviral treatment and (b) an evidence synthesis on experiences of HIVST and in-depth perspectives of the factors that facilitate or hinder HIVST uptake among adults in Africa. Initial steps towards the development of the intervention were guided by existing literature on HIVST and findings from the systematic review (**Chapter Three**) and evidence synthesis (**Chapter Four**). The findings of this initial step identified the relevant factors that facilitate or hinder HIVST uptake, provided the rationale for undertaking the project and the decision to develop a theory-based behaviour change intervention (BCI) for FBWs and MCPs in Northern Tanzania.

6.2.2 Phase 2: Identifying behavioral or environmental determinants

A formative study was conducted to explore key informants' understanding about the motivation and beliefs of the community towards HIVST and target populations'

Key informants were included in the formative study to get their perspectives on the environmental and social context towards HIVST for the target population in the study setting. Representatives of the target population provided their attitudes, beliefs, social norms, personal agency, barriers to and facilitators for HIVST uptake and linkage to HIV prevention, care and treatment.

The purpose of conducting the formative study was to gather key informants' and target populations' in-depth perspectives related to HIVST to develop a feasible, acceptable and potentially effective and sustainable BCI. Typically, both quantitative and qualitative research methods would be appropriate. However, in this project, qualitative research methods alone were conducted. Quantitative research was not possible because of limited funding. In addition, the decision to use qualitative research was influenced by the fact that HIV testing is a sensitive topic and HIVST is regarded as a 'new phenomenon' in Tanzania, so a comprehensive qualitative exploration would be valuable (Wejnert 2002). Examples of predisposing factors identified included fear of positive results, perceived adverse effects of post HIVST testing, perceived high cost of buying the test kits and fear of seeing blood/ and needle pricks. Examples of enabling factors included availability of HIVST kits and skills on how to perform the HIVST. Examples of reinforcing factors included knowledge of benefits of HIVST, knowledge of the importance of confirmatory testing after HIVST (those with preliminary reactive results) and availability of HIV prevention (male circumcision and family planning).

6.2.3 Phase 3: Educational and ecological assessment

In phase 3 of this project, the focus was to combine the key specific beliefs, barriers and enablers/facilitators, grouped by IBM constructs and to identify components and potential behaviour change techniques (BCTs) for the BCI. Mapping of the key specific beliefs, barriers and enablers/facilitators, grouped by IBM constructs for behaviour change identified in phase 2 was conducted using various behavioural change techniques (BCT). The aim was to select components of BCTs using the behaviour change technique taxonomy (BCTTv1) and intervention functions using the Behaviour Change Wheel [BCW] (Michie et al., 2011). The BCW is a theoretically driven framework based on 19 behaviour change models of health behaviour designed to enable a systematic development of interventions to support behaviour change (Michie et al., 2011). Three layers make up the 'COM-B model, which underpin the wheel. The 'Capacity' (psychological/physical) is placed at the centre, then 'Opportunity' (physical/social) and 'Motivation' (reflective/automatic). The model helps to identify which psychological determinants to address to achieve behaviour change. The second layer of the BCW is

Examples are 'education' and 'persuasion'. The third layer comprises of the policy categories, which can be used to support the delivery of the intervention functions (Michie et al., 2011).

The BCTTv1 includes 93 irreducible, discrete, hierarchically clustered and theory-linked BCTs developed to standardize the reporting of potentially active intervention elements, with extensive application in different settings. A BCT is the minutest intervention component that may have the potential to change behaviour. In addition, each intervention function is possible to consist of several BCT and one BCT may serve several functions. For instance, the BCT to instruct how to perform the behaviour may serve the intervention function of 'education' and/or 'training', contingent on the social contest and specific message (Abraham and Michie 2008, Michie et al., 2013).

In the first step, two reviewers independently mapped key specific beliefs, barriers and enablers/facilitators identified in the formative study (**Chapter Five**), grouped by IBM constructs that best explain HIVST uptake. Because 93 BCTs are likely to be difficult to work with, in step 2, the two reviewers started with a minimum set composed of 22 frequently occurring BCTs in the behavioural science literature from the BCTTv1 taxonomy (Abraham and Michie 2008, Michie et al., 2013). The decision was made as reviewing all 93 BCTs were not feasible within the proposed duration of the study. The two reviewers mapped the identified modifiable barriers and enablers/facilitators for HIVST uptake, to appropriate BCTs using the behaviour change wheel (BCW) framework developed by Michie et al. (Michie et al., 2011). The BCW links BCTs to nine intervention functions and the theoretical domains from the Theoretical Domains Framework (TDF). The TDF is a comprehensive framework of 14 theoretical domains derived from 33 behaviour change theories and 128 constructs, developed using experts consensus and validated to identify set of theoretical domains to assist in the development of BCIs (Michie et al., 2011).

In step 3, the two reviewers compared their respective matrices and used consensus between them about which BCTs were likely to be most salient. Finally, eight (8) out of 22 BCTs were selected. The consensus between the two reviewers was an attempt to approximate an objective standard of 'validity'. The eight selected BCTs are summarized in QVWŽÄÏËHĀ presented at the end of this section. Also, the two reviewers selected three (3) intervention functions from a list of nine intervention functions included in the BCW. The three (3) intervention functions were (a) education, (b) training and (c) enablement (Michie et al., 2011).Ā

Local stakeholders meeting

A stakeholders' meeting was convened with representatives from a local community advisory board (CAB). Fifteen community members attended a one-day meeting including representatives from the municipal department of health (n=2), community health workers (n= 3), HIV counsellors (n=2), people living with HIV (n=3), youth groups (n=3) and tour guides (n=2). The outline of the intervention was presented and feedback was sought on appropriate session length, mode of delivery and on social and cultural acceptance of the components of the proposed intervention. The members used their expertise and experiences to consider the practicability of delivery of the components of the intervention in the study setting. Discussions during the workshop elicited concrete feedback, which was used to modify the contents of the intervention.

For example, the stakeholders recommended ***"Wawezeshaji rika"-*** a Swahili word for peer educators (PEs). In addition, stakeholders suggested that training topics for peer educators should cover the following: (a) perceived barriers to/facilitators for HIVST uptake (b) myths around the use of HIVST uptake (c) self-confidence towards HIVST uptake (d) positive and negative consequences of HIVST uptake and (e) skills on using Oral Quick HIVST test kits. Stakeholders mentioned the roles and responsibilities of PEs as follows: (a) to provide correct information to the participants (b) to make a proper follow-up of participants according to the study protocol (c) to keep all participants' personal information confidential and (d) to show respect to participants throughout the study. Roles and responsibilities of the participants were to (a) be respectful to PEs and other participants (b) be cooperative throughout the study (c) be fully engaged during the training and (d) keep all participants' personal information confidential. Finally, stakeholders mentioned challenges for the implementation of the HIVST that should be addressed as (a) fear of participants being seen by others while carrying the HIVST test kits in public (b) the English language used in the information package for instruction on how to use the HIVST test kits and (c) the sensitivity and privacy associated with HIV testing. It was recommended that dark envelopes should be used to carry the HIVST self-test kits, a Swahili version for instruction on how to use the HIVST test kits should be available for participants and the intervention should be delivered on a 'one-on-one' format as opposed to a group format.

6.2.4 Phase 4: Developing the BCI

In phase 4 of this book, described in the present chapter, a workbook was designed to assist the trained peer-educators to implement the BCI. The workbook used BCTs to regulate negative feelings associated with receiving positive HIV test results, fear of

Other BCTs incorporated in the workbook focused on the social consequences of performing or not performing HIVST, beliefs of significant others about the target population's HIV testing behaviours and their approval of using HIVST.

Emphasis was put on the past success of life experiences of target populations rather than on failure to enable behaviour change. The trained PEs used the workbook during the two sessions of the BCI delivered over 2 days.

From the implementation science, the study identified mass media and motivational interviewing (MI) techniques through peer-education by trained opinion leaders (OLs) as key strategies that could directly facilitate the BCI to increase HIVST uptake. The MI technique is a client-centred approach used to enhance the client's internal motivation to change by exploring and solving their uncertainty (Rollnick and Miller 1995). In brief, the MI technique is based on four major strategies as follows (a) expressing empathy - an understanding and acceptance of the participant's knowledge, attitudes and experiences rather than trainer's role as an expert; (b) developing discrepancy between the participant's current and desired behaviour (i.e. between the current situation and what a person needs); (c) rolling with resistance and not against it to prevent communication rupture and allowing participants to explore their views towards the behaviour (e.g. HIVST) and (d) supporting self-efficacy (i.e. the confidence in their ability to change/or perform the behaviour) (Rollnick and Miller 1995). Guided by the diffusion of innovation theory (DIT), the study used opinion leaders (OLs) - persons who influence the opinions, attitudes, beliefs, motivations and behaviours of their peers. The DIT has been successfully applied in different settings in using opinion leaders as agents of behaviour change (Valente and Pumpuang 2007). This project did not focus on the macro level, but the micro-level, as described below.

In phase 4 of this project, the focus was to align the component of the intervention, intervention functions and the BCTs at the micro-level to develop an engaging and informative BCI tailored for FBWs and MCPs. The content of session 1 focused on perceived norms and beliefs about HIVST. The goals of session 1 were to alleviate negative feelings about fears associated with HIVST, decrease perceptions of barriers related to HIVST, reinforce enablers for HIVST, correct misconceptions about HIVST and reinforce subjective and descriptive norms associated with HIVST uptake. The BCTs for session 1 include regulation of negative emotions, information about social consequences, information about others' approval and focus on past success.

The content of session 2 focused on HIVST knowledge and skills on the use of self-test kits. The goals of session 2 were to increase knowledge of HIVST, build confidence and skills to use HIV self-test kits and to provide feedback to participants on their performance in using the self-test kits. The BCTs for session 2 included instruction on how to perform the behaviour, demonstration of the behaviour, prompt for practice and feedback on outcome of behaviour.

Once the content and structure of the workbook were finalized, mass-media materials (i.e. photographic materials, leaflets and video) were compiled. The resources included photographic materials and interactive cards and a take-home leaflet. The materials focused on knowledge about HIVST, benefits of HIVST, barriers for HIVST, perceived myths related with using HIVST, sources of social support e.g. significant others' approval of using HIVST, and perceived confidence and skills to conduct HIVST alone in privacy. The take-home leaflet was a copy of the pictorial instructions on how to do HIVST in Swahili, meant for reinforcement of the information delivered in the sessions (Table 6.1).

To engage OLs to promote the uptake of HIVST, 10 most frequently mentioned participants (MCPs =5; FBWs = 5), were invited and trained to become peer-educators (PEs). Potential OLs were those whose advice or encouragement was sought by peers when making health decisions. A sample socio-metric method (Constenbader and Valente 2003) was used to identify, select and recruit the opinion leaders. The OLs had the advantage of being able to spend more time with their peers, who were likely to feel more comfortable with them in discussing a sensitive topic such as HIVST

Opinion leadership workshop

Opinion leaders attended two full-day training sessions conducted by the candidate [BN], to become peer-educators (PEs). The training comprised of addressing the roles and responsibilities of a peer educator, routes of HIV transmission to alleviate HIV misconceptions, and skills on the appropriate use of oral-fluid HIVST kits including a live demonstration and simulation on how to use the kits. The content of HIVST kits uses including the importance of confirmatory blood-based HIV testing for all self-testers reporting reactive test results or prevention strategies such as voluntary medical male circumcision or family planning for those reporting negative test results. Throughout the training, OLs also learned effective communication strategy (i.e. motivational interviewing technique), including how to counter negative viewpoints.

Skill-building using participatory methods was a major component of the training. It involved role-playing delivery of the intervention sessions in Swahili, methods to engage peers in conversations about the BCI and how to improve PEs listening skills. A modest allowance was given to attendees to cover transportation costs to and from the training venue. An attendance register was used to record attendance.

The trained PEs provided the BCI to increase HIVST uptake and linkage to HIV prevention, care and treatment among their peers for a period of one month. PEs helped participants to moderate their negative feelings about fears of positive results, adverse effects of post HIVST testing and fear of seeing blood and/or needle pricks. For example, the use of oral HIVST tests was introduced as a measure to alleviate the fear of seeing blood or receiving a needle prick. PEs also informed peers about the benefits of HIV testing in general and HIVST in particular, the importance of confirmatory testing after HIVST (i.e. those reporting a reactive result) and HIV prevention strategies (e.g. male circumcision and family planning services). The PEs highlighted social consequences related to not performing (e.g. being infected with HIV) or performing HIVST (e.g. fear of HIV positive results) and emphasized on significant others' (e.g. parents, peers, relatives, friends, etc.) approval of using HIVST. The PEs used an educational strategy (i.e. adapted motivational interviewing (MI) technique) to deliver the BCI. Based on the MI technique, trained PEs carried out the sessions, which were approximately 45 to 60 minutes, in a simple and clear Swahili, to foster discussions and allow questions from participants rather than provide prescriptive, unequivocal and unidirectional information.

Table 6.1. IBM constructs, intervention functions, Behavioural Change Techniques and application

IBM constructs	Description of what needs addressing in the Intervention based on formative research/ literature	Intervention Functions	Behavioural Change Techniques (BCTs) identified	Application
Experiential attitudes	• Fear of positive test result • Fear of adverse effects post HIVST testing • Fear of seeing blood/ and needle pricks	• Education*	**11.2.** Regulate negative emotions	**11:2.** Peer-educators help participants to moderate negative feelings about fear of positive results, adverse effects post HIVST testing and fear of seeing blood/and needle pricks, with alternative positive thoughts or situational role reversal (e.g., use of oral HIVST tests).
Instrumental attitudes	• A lack of knowledge about the benefits of HIVST-knowledge about what it does, what it offers beyond what people may already know, etc.	• Education* • Training**	**4:1.** Instruction on how to perform the behaviour **5:3** Information about social consequences **6:3** Information about others' approval	
Perceived norms	• Peers/co-workers support • Encouragement from opinion leaders	• Education* • Training**	**4:1** Instruction on how to perform the behaviour **6:1** Demonstration of the behaviour **6:3** Information about others' approval	**4:1.** Descriptions on how to use the HIVST test kits were provided to participants.
Perceived control	• Potential to minimize stigma and/or discrimination • The perception that the cost of HIVST kits is a	• Education* • Training** Enablement***	**2:7** Feedback on the outcome(s) **4:1** Instruction on how to perform the behaviour **6:1** Demonstration of the behaviour	**5:3.** Peer educators provide information about the benefits of HIVST and advantages of testing or disadvantages of

	barrier-low or free HIVST kits may increase uptake. • The perception that poverty, residing in rural settings and physical disabilities are barriers to HIV testing • Effective communication channels • Autonomy to test for HIV • Opportunity to test for HIV.		success **11.2.** Regulate negative emotions	HIV, focusing on the social consequences if the person does or does not perform the HIVST. **6:3.** Peer-educators provide about what significant others (e.g., parents, peers, relatives, friends, etc.) think about the person's HIV testing behaviour and emphasize significant other's approve of using HIVST.
Self-efficacy	• Availability of in-person counselling. • Correct information will clear doubts about an individual's capacity to perform HIVST • Less confidence to	• Education* • Training** Enablement***	**2:7** Feedback on outcome(s) behaviour **4:1** Instruction on how to perform the behaviour **6:1** Demonstration of the behaviour **8:1** Prompt	**2:7.** Peer-educators providing feedback to participants on how they performed on how to use the HIV self-testing. **6:1.** Peer-educators showed a 5-minutes video on how to use an oral-based HIV test

			success.	**8:1.** Peer-educators ask the person to rehearse HIV self-testing after viewing the video. **15:3.** Peer-educators help the person to focus on the past success of life experience rather than on failures.
*Increasing knowledge or understanding ** Imparting skills ***Increasing means/reducing barriers to increase capacity beyond education and training.				

6.3 Discussion

This chapter describes the development of a theory-based Behaviour Change Intervention (BCI) for FBWs and MCPs to increase HIVST uptake and linkage to HIV prevention, care and treatment in Northern Tanzania. The process included extensive systematic review and evidence synthesis, formative research among key informants and the target population and the application of the IBM and the PRECEDE-PROCEED planning model. This chapter illustrates a systematic, theory and evidence-informed approach to developing an intervention that aimed to improve the uptake of HIV testing among hard to reach populations. The PRECEDE - PROCEED model as a 'road map' guided the development of the intervention as described in this chapter. Using the PRECEDE -PROCEED model enhanced the likelihood of the BCI being effective, acceptable to the targeted population and feasible to implement (Green and Kreuter 1999).

The inclusion of each process that was undertaken in the development of the intervention ensured that the intervention was founded on theory and evidence. The components of the intervention addressed the identified key beliefs, facilitators/ and potential barriers guided by IBM that best explained the uptake of HIV testing. Further, the alignment process helped to tailor the components of the intervention to suit the social context of the local setting.

The systematic use of the BCTs approach assisted in the selection of intervention functions and specific BCTs from the BCCTv1 (Abraham and Michie 2008, Michie et al., 2013). The result was the selection of relevant BCTs and intervention functions likely to initiate behavioural change logically and transparently.

This intervention was built upon the IBM theory but required adaptation and tailoring to the specific needs of the target population. Findings from the formative research highlighted the use of existing social networks of the targeted population, particularly MCPs, as an effective strategy to promote awareness for HIV testing.

A similar finding was reported from a study conducted in Dar es Salaam among men from stable social networks, which observed that their acceptability of HIVST intervention might be possible through opinion leadership (Conserve et al., 2016, Maman et al., 2016, Conserve et al., 2018, Conserve et al., 2018).

To create awareness and buy into the idea of the intervention, this project conducted a multidisciplinary stakeholders meeting. Stakeholders' inputs included discussions on the nomination process of 'opinion leaders' who were trained to provide the BCI, which targeted attitudes, beliefs and personal agency of the target population. During the meeting, stakeholders discussed the key roles and responsibilities of the trained opinion leaders (i.e. peer-educators). The suggested roles and responsibilities included the provision of correct information to the trainees, proper follow-up of trainees, maintaining the confidentiality of trainees' information and showing respect to fellow PEs and trainees. Existing evidence suggests that opinion leadership is used in health-related interventions to gain support for and implementation of community health-related interventions (Valente and Pumpuang 2007).

Another adaptation of the intervention was the use of an effective communication channel based upon an educational strategy, the motivational interviewing (MI) technique. Findings from the formative research and inputs from the stakeholders meeting suggested that effective communication channels would be imperative in creating awareness, advocacy and promotion of the intervention. MI technique is built upon the Prochaska's stage of change, which suggests that behavioural change is a complex and cyclical process, involving interactions between physical dependence, social factors and motivation. This description helps to refute the concept that behaviour change is a straightforward decision to change based on information about the health risks (Prochaska et al., 1994).

Opinion leaders were trained on the basic principles of the MI technique to stimulate intrinsic motivation (e.g. decision to test for HIV) of the study participants. Further, opinion leaders were asked to encourage participants to explore their uncertainty about HIVST testing and their readiness to change.

Also, PEs were trained to create a good rapport by avoiding arguments, discussing stigmatized behaviours, expressing empathy (i.e. acceptance of the participants' knowledge, attitudes and experiences of HIV testing) and to acknowledge participants' autonomy in deciding to test for, or not to test for HIV.

The process and outcomes of the BCI were evaluated 3 months post-intervention, using a before-after study design. The process evaluation involved an assessment of the acceptability, feasibility and fidelity of the BCI, whilst the outcome evaluation assessed the effect of the BCI on HIVST uptake and linkage to HIV prevention, care and treatment.

However, a randomized clinical trial (RCT) would have been the most ideal study design to evaluate the effectiveness of the BCI to change HIV testing behaviour of the target population. The before - after study design was selected as an alternative because it is cheaper and easier to conduct and will yield evidence closer to a cluster-randomized trial. The details of the process and outcome evaluations are reported in **Chapter Seven**.

6.4 Conclusion

This chapter described the design and development of a theory-based BCI for FBWs and MCPs to increase HIVST uptake and linkage to HIV prevention, care and treatment in Northern Tanzania. From a conceptual perspective, this intervention, which was based on IBM theory, using a planning model (PRECEDE-PROCEED) and implementation strategies described above, was feasible, acceptable and effective at increasing the uptake of HIV testing. Existing evidence supports the effectiveness of theory-based BCIs to HIV/STI prevention globally (van Empelen et al., 2003, Wolfers et al., 2007, Mkumbo et al., 2009, Corbie-Smith et al., 2010, Wolfers et al., 2012, Theunissen et al., 2013, Aarø et al., 2016). However, to the author's knowledge, there is no evidence of a BCI developed for FBWs and MCPs in this setting.

The strength of this intervention and the process used was the documentation of decisions throughout the selection process of intervention components robustly and transparently.

This approach provided a deeper understanding and insight into the relevant intervention components, which enabled the development of a tailored, theory-based BCI. Hence, the process and outcome evaluations of this intervention will add to the evidence of the acceptability and feasibility of a theory-based BCI to increase HIVST uptake and linkage to HIV prevention, care and treatment. However, using a before-after study design, instead of a RCT to evaluate whether the robust process led to measurable effectiveness may be a limitation.

In future, evaluation of a BCI of this nature should consider using an RCT to evaluate the impact of the BCI on attitudes, beliefs, personal agency and behaviours of the target population and factors thought to mediate the effect of the intervention along causal pathways of change (Garba and Gadanya 2017).

Should such a future RCT intervention prove efficacious, it will allow scaling up of HIVST use in this study setting. A potential methodological limitation of this study could be the influence of how the research team operationalized the theoretical domains in terms of appropriate intervention components. For this intervention, only one research team conducted the systematic and replicable process, which is a limitation. Interventionists need to understand how best to operationalize theory in the context of intervention development, selection and designing intervention components.

6.5 Lessons learned

The design process described in this chapter provided some key lessons for the development of a theory-based BCI for the target populations (a) the importance of extensive systematic reviews and evidence synthesis, formative research and stakeholders inputs to adapt and tailor behaviours theories domains to address

(b) the importance of drawing upon multiple theories in designing an intervention that was perceived highly feasible within the study setting and (c) the acceptability of using trained PEs for delivery of a theory-based BCI, with appropriate training and supervision.

References

Aarø, L. E., A. J. Flisher, S. Kaaya, H. Onya, M. Fuglesang, K. Klepp, et al. (2016). "Promoting sexual and reproductive health in early adolescence in South Africa and Tanzania: Development of a theory- and evidence-based intervention programme." Scandinavian Journal of Public Health **34**(2): 150-158.

Abraham, C. and S. Michie (2008). "A taxonomy of behavior change techniques used in interventions." Health Psychology **27**(3): 379-387.

Azjen, I. (2006). "Constructing a TPB Questionnaire: Conceptual and Methodological Considerations." Retrieved 12/1/2014, 2014, from http://www.people.umass.edu/aizen/pdf/tbp.measurement.pdf.

Bandura, A. (2004). "Health promotion by social cognitive means." Health Educ Behav **31**(2): 143-164.

Bartholomew, L. K., G. S. Parcel, G. Kok, N. H. Gottlieb and M. E. Fernández (2011). Planning Health Promotion Programs: An Intervention Mapping Approach, Jossy-Bass.

Conserve, D., L. Kajula, T. Yamanis and S. Maman (2016). "Formative Research to Develop Human Immunodeficiency Virus (HIV) Self-Testing Intervention Among Networks of Men in Dar es Salaam, Tanzania: A Mixed Methods Approach." Open Forum Infectious Diseases, Volume 3, Issue suppl_1, **3**,(1,): 518.

Conserve, D. F., D. Alemu, T. Yamanis, S. Maman and L. Kajula (2018). "He Told Me to Check My Health":
A Qualitative Exploration of Social Network Influence on Men's HIV Testing Behavior and HIV Self-Testing Willingness in Tanzania." American Journal of Men's Health.

Conserve, D. F., K. E. Muessig, L. L. Maboko, S. Shirima, M. N. Kilonzo, S. Maman, et al. (2018). "Mate Yako Afya Yako: Formative research to develop the Tanzania HIV self-testing education and promotion (Tanzania STEP) project for men." PLoS ONE.

Constenbader, E. and T. W. Valente (2003). "The stability of centrality measures when networks are sampled." Social Networks **25**: 283-307.

Corbie-Smith, G., A. Akers, C. Blumenthal, B. Council, M. Wynn, M. Muhammad, et al. (2010). "Intervention mapping as a participatory approach to developing an HIV prevention intervention in rural African American communities." AIDS Education and Prevention **22**(3): 184-202.

Fishbein, M. (2007). A Reasoned Action Approach:Some Issues, Questions, a nd Clarifications. Prediction and Change of Health Behaviour: Applying the Reasoned Action Approach. I. Ajzen, D.Albaraccin and R.Hornik., Hillsdale,N .J.:E rlbaum,2007.

Fishbein, M. and I. Azjen (1975). Belief,A ttitude,I ntention, and Behaviour:A n Introduction to Theory and Research., Reading,M ass.: A ddison-Wesley.

Garba, R. M. and M. A. Gadanya (2017). "The role of intervention mapping in designing disease prevention interventions: A systematic review of the literature." PLoS ONE **12**(3): e0174438.

Glanz, K., B. K. Rimer and K. Viswanath (2008). Health behavior and health education:theory, research, and practice. San Francisco, Jossey-Bass.

Godin, G., A. Belanger-Gravel, M. Eccles and J. Grimshaw (2008). "Healthcare professional's intentions and behaviours: A systematic review of studies based on social cognitive theories." Implementation Science **3**(36): 1-12.

Green.L.W. and M. W. Kreuter (1999). Health Promotion and Planning: An educational and ecological approach. Mayfield: Moutain View, CA.

Hoffmann, T. C., P. P. Glasziou, I. Boutron, R. Milne, R. Perera, D. Moher, et al. (2014). "Better reporting of interventions: template for intervention description and replication (TIDieR) checklist and guide." BMJ **348**: g1687.

Maman, S., L. Kajula, P. Balvanz, M. Kilonzo, M. Mulawa and T. Yamanis (2016). "Leveraging strong social ties among young men in Dar es Salaam: A pilot intervention of microfinance and peer leadership for HIV and gender-based violence prevention." Glob Public Health **11**(10): 1202-1215.

Michie, S., M. Richardson, M. Johnston, C. Abraham, J. Francis, W. Hardeman, et al. (2013). "The behavior change technique taxonomy (v1) of 93 hierarchically clustered techniques: building an international consensus for the reporting of behavior change interventions." Annals of Behaviour Medicine **46**(1): 81-95.

Michie, S., M. M. van Stralen and R. West (2011). "The behaviour change wheel: A new method for characterizing and designing behaviour change interventions." Implementation Science **6**(42): 1-11.

Mkumbo, K., H. Schaalma, S. Kaaya, J. Leerlooijer, J. Mbwambo and G. Kilonzo (2009). "The application of Intervention Mapping in developing and implementing school-based sexuality and HIV/AIDS education in a developing country context: the case of Tanzania." Scandinavian Journal of Public Health **37 Suppl 2**: 28-36.

Mokdad, A. H., W. H. Giles, B. A. Bowman, G. A. Mensah, E. S. Ford, S. M. Smith, et al. (2004). "Changes in health behaviors among older Americans, 1990 to 2000." Public Health Report **119**(3): 356-361.

Prochaska, J. O., C. A. Redding, L. L. Harlow, J. S. Rossi and W. F. Velicer (1994). "The Transtheoretical Model of Change and HIV Prevention: A Review." Health Education Quarterly **Vol. 21**((4):): 471-486

Rollnick, S. and W. R. Miller (1995). "What is motivational interviewing?" Behavioural and Cognitive Psychotherapy **23**: 325-334.

Theunissen, K. A., C. J. Hoebe, R. Crutzen, C. Kara-Zaïtri, N. K. de Vries, J. E. van Bergen, et al. (2013). "Using intervention mapping for the development of a targeted secure web-based outreach strategy named SafeFriend, for Chlamydia trachomatis testing in young people at risk." BMC Public Health **13**(996).

Valente, T. W. and P. Pumpuang (2007). "Identifying opinion leaders to promote behavior change." Health Education & Behavior **34**(6): 881-896.

van Empelen, P., G. Kok, H. P. Schaalma and L. K. Bartholomew (2003). "An AIDS risk reduction program for Dutch drug users: an intervention mapping approach to planning. ." Health Promotion Practice **4** (4): 402–412

Wejnert, B. (2002). "Integrating Models of Diffusion of Innovations: A Conceptual Framework." Annual Review of Sociology **28**: 297-326.

Wolfers, M., O. de Zwart and G. Kok (2012). "The systematic development of ROsafe: an intervention to promote STI testing among vocational school students." Health Promotion Practice **13**(3): 378–387

Wolfers, M. E., C. van den Hoek, J. Brug and O. de Zwart (2007). "Using Intervention Mapping to develop a programme to prevent sexually transmittable infections, including HIV, among heterosexual migrant men." BMC Public Health **7**: 141.

Ā

Ā

CHAPTER SEVEN

7.0 Evaluation of a theory-based behaviour change intervention to increase HIVST uptake and linkage to HIV prevention, care and treatment among Female Bar Workers and Male Mountain Climbing Porters in Northern Tanzania.

7.1 Introduction

The UNAIDS has declared global targets of 95-95-95 which states that 5 % of people living with HIV being aware of their HIV status; 95% of those living with HIV are on Anti-retroviral treatment (ART) and 95% of those on ART achieve viral suppression by 2030 ·(UNAIDS 2018). To achieve these ambitious UNAIDS global targets; people must know their HIV status through HIV Testing Services (HTS). Evidence has shown that HTS is an essential component of HIV control programmes and an entry point of HIV care, treatment and support services (UNAIDS 2017). Early detection, initiation of treatment and care and introduction of risk reduction strategies are major benefits associated with HTS (UNAIDS/WHO 2010, Wanyenze et al., 2011, UNAIDS 2014, UNAIDS 2017, UNAIDS 2019).

Even with these benefits and the wider availability of HTS options and ART for HIV-infected patients, testing rates remain low in sub-Saharan Africa (SSA) (Staveteig et al., 2013). The low rates of HTS uptake in SSA are inextricably linked with stigma and discrimination related to an HIV positive result (Mukolo et al., 2013, Njau et al., 2014, Ostermann et al., 2014). Health system barriers contributing to the limited uptake, particularly in clinical settings include fear of visibility, lack of confidentiality of HIV positive test result (Mukolo et al., 2013), a lack of privacy and waiting time to obtain a test result (Musheke et al., 2013). Other, health system barriers associated with low uptake include lack of human or technical resources (i.e., counsellors, or HIV testing reagents), long queues at HIV testing points and inconvenient hours of operation (Morin et al., 2006, Negin et al., 2009, Ahmed et al., 2013).

Furthermore, there are gender differentials in HIV testing uptake in SSA, with more women compared to men aware of their HIV status. Evidence shows that the uptake of HIV testing ranges between 1% and 42 % among women, while for men it ranges between 2 % and 38% (Staveteig et al., 2013).

A similar scenario of gender differentials in HIV testing rates is reported in Tanzania. According to the 2016-2017 Tanzania HIV Impact Survey (THIS), only 45 % of men compared to 55 % of women were aware of their HIV status. Of significance, among men living with HIV who have tested for HIV, 86% reported initiation of ART, of whom 84% reported viral suppression (THIS 2017).

Several barriers explain men' reluctance to test for HIV, the key of which are their masculinity ideals, which prevent them from expressing emotions in public (Njau et al., 2012, Morfaw et al., 2013, Kumwenda et al., 2014, Choko et al., 2017, Choko et al., 2017, Matovu et al., 2018). Another barrier, is the perception that HIV testing is a woman's domain (Conserve et al., 2018a, Conserve et al., 2018b). Besides, perceived sense of risk related to extramarital affairs and the resultant fear of receiving a positive diagnosis and limited time to visit HIV testing points exacerbating men's reluctance to test for HIV (Njau et al., 2012, Mukolo et al., 2013, Musheke et al., 2013, The IeDEA and ART cohort collaborations 2014, Conserve et al., 2018a, Conserve et al., 2018b). Among women, fear of potential conflicts that may arise following a positive HIV test, particularly in unstable relationships marked by distrust may be a barrier for HIV testing (Njau et al., 2012). Other barriers for poor uptake of HIV testing among women include the low perceived risk of being infected with HIV because they trust their male partners, fear of visibility while visiting a testing centre, which is related with sexual promiscuity and assumed HIV- positive status and abstaining from sex or lacking a sexual partner (Musheke et al., 2013).

Such barriers limit progress towards the UNAIDS 95-95-95 global targets by 2030 and calls for universal scaling up of HTS (UNAIDS 2017). Complementing existing HTS approaches with novel testing methods such as HIVST might overcome or circumvent some of the barriers to HIV testing. (WHO 2016)

Studies from Kenya (Kalibala et al., 2014, Thirumurthy et al., 2016), Malawi (Choko et al., 2015), Nigeria (Brown et al., 2015), Uganda (Asiimwe et al., 2014), Tanzania (Conserve et al., 2016, Jennings et al., 2017), DRC (Tonen-Wolyec et al., 2018) and South Africa (Pant Pai et al., 2013, Makusha et al., 2015, Mokgatle and Madiba 2017), have demonstrated high acceptability and uptake of HIVST in SSA (Krause et al., 2013).

These studies have also shown that HIVST interventions may be effective in increasing uptake of HIV testing in the general population, among young people and key populations (Spielberg et al., 2004, Cambiano et al., 2015, WHO 2015, Neuman et al., 2018, Hatzold et al., 2019).

In 2012, the US Food and Drug Administration approved the oral HIVST, (US Food and Drug Administration(FDA) 2012) and in 2015, oral HIVST was authorized in Europe (Prazuck et al., 2016). In low-income countries, including African countries, regulated HIVST kits are not yet available for the general population (WHO & UNITAID 2016). In December 2016, the World Health Organization (WHO) formally recommended HIVST as an additional option to HTS (WHO 2016) and to develop and validate HIVST (WHO 2016).

Despite existing WHO HIVST guidelines and technical recommendations that highlight the potential contribution of HIVST to close gaps in universal HIV testing coverage, most SSA countries, including Tanzania have lagged in the adoption of HIVST (WHO 2016). HIV policymakers, HIV experts and government stakeholders in many African countries have expressed several concerns, challenges and criticism related to HIVST (Makusha et al., 2015, van Rooyen et al., 2015). The main concerns against HIVST include potential psychological and social harms due to lack of face-to-face counselling, risks of inaccurate results and uncertainty over linkage to care for individuals with a reactive HIVST test result (Mavedzenge et al., 2013, Makusha et al., 2015, van Rooyen et al., 2015, Gagnon et al., 2018). However, some of the concerns about HIVST, such as the potential of psychological and social harms are not yet supported with evidence (Gagnon et al., 2018).

In Tanzania, HIVST is recognized as a potential testing option to increase HIV testing rates for high-risk populations (TACAIDS 2018). Also, the National AIDS control programme (NACP) is preparing an HIVST guideline, to assist potential users to access HIV care treatment and support including confirmatory tests, initiation of ART and PrePEP (Conserve et al., 2018). As of July 2018, Tanzania's National HIV Testing Guidelines did not allow HIVST. However, at the time of writing, plans were underway to change the law to allow the use of HIVST. Further changes are expected on the introduction of HIVST into the national HTS policy, which will be informed by findings from ongoing studies among key populations in selected regions with high HIV prevalence in the country (TACAIDS 2018).

Implementation science suggests that behaviour change interventions (BCIs) grounded on theories are effective at individual, community and population levels (Davis et al., 2015, Villalobos et al., 2019). However, the effectiveness of BCIs are relatively modest with considerable heterogeneity of short-term and long-term effects. Besides, ineffective interventions do exist in implementation science literature (Michie et al., 2013). Additionally, there is a dearth of information related to fidelity of implementation of BCI in the implementation of science literature (Davis et al., 2015, Villalobos et al., 2019). The query as to whether BCI that are overtly grounded on theory are more effective than those that are not is complex (Davis et al., 2015). One key factor that may explain the query is the poor application of theory (Davis et al., 2015, Villalobos et al., 2019).

There is a lack of information on the links between behaviour change techniques and theoretical constructs in most theory-based interventions, or whether all the constructs were targeted by behaviour change techniques may influence the effectiveness of the BCI (Davis et al., 2015, Villalobos Dintrans et al., 2019). An alternative explanation may be inappropriate selection of theory. An appropriate theory that is effective to bring about a specific behaviour change is very important to bring about the expected behaviour change (Davis et al., 2015, Villalobos et al., 2019). To circumvent this fundamental limitation described above, this book adopted the

At present, there is a dearth of information on the acceptability and feasibility of a behaviour change interventions (BCIs) to increase HIVST uptake and linkage to HIV prevention, care and treatment among FBWs and MCPs in Tanzania.

It is important to generate information on the acceptability and feasibility of a BCI to increase HIVST uptake and linkage to HIV prevention, care and treatment. This study aimed to evaluate the acceptability and feasibility of the BCI and its impact on FBWs and MCPs beliefs, attitudes and personal agency to increase HIVST uptake and linkage to HIV prevention, care and treatment in Northern Tanzania. The process evaluation sought to assess the acceptability and feasibility of the BCI and fidelity of its implementation. The outcome evaluation sought to measure the uptake of HIVST, the prevalence of HIV positive diagnoses and linkage to HIV prevention, care and treatment.

7.2 Study setting and population

The study was conducted in an urban setting in Northern Tanzania with a high HIV prevalence and low uptake of HTS. Kilimanjaro Region has a total population of 1.6 million and the average household size of 4.3 (United Republic of Tanzania 2012). The study area is in the tourist circuit, with major national parks as well as the highest mountain in Africa, Mt. Kilimanjaro.

Most tourist hotels and bars are located in northern Tanzania. An HIV prevalence report of eight regions in the country, including two in northern Tanzania (Kilimanjaro and Arusha), witnessed an increase in prevalence, despite the overall decline in national HIV prevalence. For example, HIV prevalence increased from 1.9% in 2007/08 to 3.8 % in 2011/12 in the Kilimanjaro region. Moshi Municipal Council is among seven (7) districts in Kilimanjaro region of Tanzania. Other six districts are Rombo, Mwanga, Same, Moshi rural, Hai and Siha District Councils. Moshi Municipal Council has an estimated population of 184,292 in 21 ward administrative units, with an average household size of 4.0 (United Republic of Tanzania 2012).

At the time of data collection, 18 facilities were providing HTS. Also, 21 HIV care and treatment centres (CTC) provide access to antiretroviral therapy (ART), in the study setting (Ostermann et al., 2014).
The study population comprised FBWs and MCPs in Kilimanjaro region. It is estimated that 2,000 young women between the ages of 18 and 40 years work in more than 600 licensed establishments, with additional FBWs working in unlicensed alcohol selling venues in the study setting. In the study setting, HIV prevalence among FBWs is proportionally higher (19% to 26%) than in the general population (5.1%) (THIS 2017).

The observed high HIV prevalence among FBWs is associated with HIV risk behaviours, such as excessive alcohol consumption, multiple sexual partnerships and transactional sexual practices (Kapiga et al., 2002, Ao et al., 2006). Although 95 % of FBWs reported previously having been tested for HIV, 41% of those who have tested have never repeated HIV testing in the past year (Ostermann et al., 2015). An estimated 17,000 porters working in the tourist industry are predominantly young men (between the ages of 18 and 45 years), who are very mobile and face volatile income cycles (Peaty 2010). According to Lyamuya et al (2017) the behaviour of MCPs puts them at risk for HIV infection. These behaviours include unprotected sex, multiple concurrent sexual partnerships, substance use, alcohol consumption and marijuana use (Lyamuya et al., 2017). Additionally, one-third of MCPs have never tested for HIV, despite engaging in high-risk behaviours for HIV infection (Ostermann et al., 2015).

7.3 Methods

7.3.1 Study design

The project used an uncontrolled before-after study design, which was deemed appropriate in achieving the study objectives. The before-after study design used a “historical” comparison in the form of the "control group". This study design aimed to compare changes in values within individual overtime, before the intervention (pre-test) and after the intervention (post-test) and not between the individual and a comparison group. The study tested the same individuals before and after the BCI. Because of the nature of the before-after design, no baseline data on outcomes of

In addition, the study measured a 'one-time point' measurement after the intervention. A minimum sample of 170 participants was estimated using a confidence interval approach (Lenth 2001). Assuming HIVST uptake of 87.2% or greater, a significance margin error (ME) of 5% and a confidence level of 95%, with 80 % power, we calculated that a sample of 170 participants were required (Choko et al., 2011).ĀThe before-after study design was conducted between March 2018 (pre-intervention phase) and July 2018 (post-intervention phase).

The baseline data was collected from all eligible participants who agreed to participate in the study before the BCI was offered to those who agreed to participate in the intervention. Participants who participated in the intervention were followed over 12 weeks (3-months) to measure the outcomes of interest.

7.3.2 Logic model for implementation

A logic model (Figure 7.1) was developed to make explicit the theoretically informed assumptions about determinants of behaviour change and how intervention strategies are assumed to affect them. The logic model consists of the description of the intervention strategies (inputs/resources), proximal outcomes (IBM constructs), process outcomes (acceptability, feasibility and fidelity of implementation) and impact outcomes (HIVST uptake, the prevalence of HIV positive diagnosis, linkage to HIV prevention, care and treatment and knowledge of HIV testing and HIVST). The logic model demonstrates the intended pathways of behaviour change from the intervention strategies, through change mechanisms (mediators), and intended process and impact outcomes guided by the Integrated Behavior Model of behaviour change.

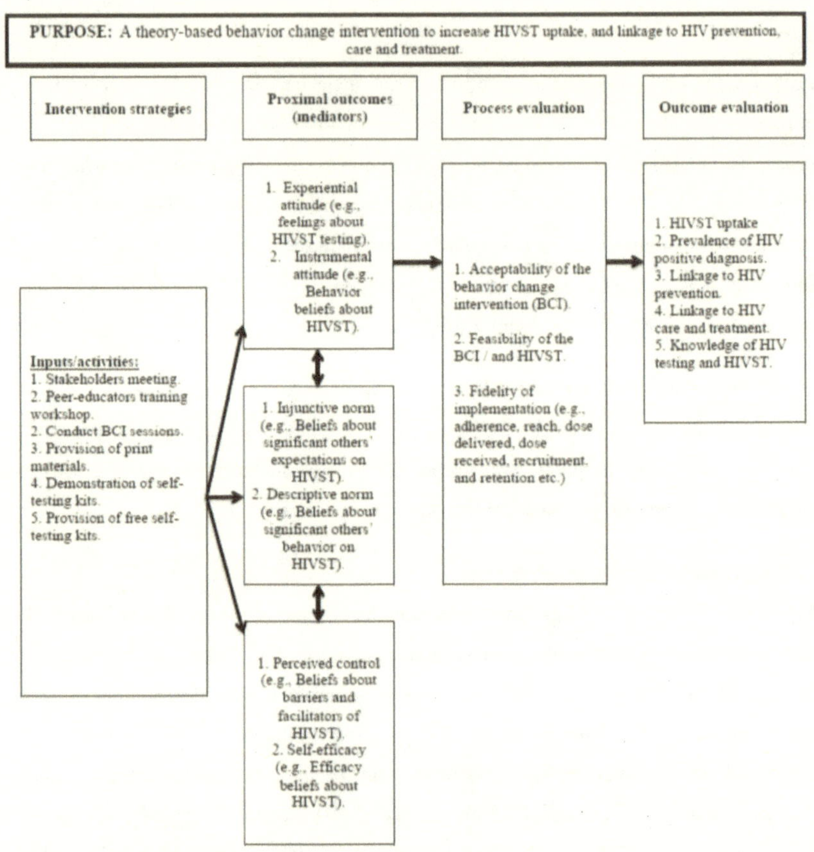

Figure 7.1. Logic model for the implementation of the IBM behaviour change intervention (Source: Logic model constructed by the author).

7.3.3 Study participants

We recruited participants who were 18 years of age or older at the time of enrolment, and who self-reported an HIV-negative status and had not had an HIV test in the past 3 months or self-reported that their HIV status was unknown. The recruitment strategy involved invitations delivered by trained peer educators (PEs) to eligible participants to visit the study office within the study setting for consenting to participate in the study. All eligible participants provided written, informed consent to participate in the study. Participants providing written consent were sent back to the trained PEs to schedule attendance at the first intervention session. Ethical approval was obtained from the Kilimanjaro Christian Medical University College Research and Ethical Reviews Committee, the National Institute of Medical Research in Tanzania, Tanzania Food and Drugs Authority and the Health Sciences Research Ethics Committee at the University of Cape Town in South Africa.

7.4 Outcomes

7.4.1 Demographics

The following demographic information was collected at baseline from eligible study participants using a semi-structured paper-based questionnaire: gender, age, marital status, level of education, religion and living arrangement.

Ā

7.4.2 Acceptability

Acceptability was assessed qualitatively from selected study participants. Feedback from participants was obtained for individual sessions (following sessions 1-2) and intervention overall (post-test follow-up). Also, 10 participants (MCPs = 5; FBWs =5) participated in exit interviews to explore their experience in participating in the intervention. The exit interviews aimed to get an insight on participant's experiences with the BCI and HIVST uptake.ĀAn in-depth interview guide was used to collect information on acceptability and feasibility of the BCI, fidelity of implementation and personal experiences of HIVST uptake.ĀĀ

Ā

Ā

7.4.3 Feasibility

Participants assessed the feasibility of the BCI at the end of session 2 by rating the intervention sessions and materials. The ratings were on intervention sessions and materials (e.g. " Overall, the contents of the sessions were understandable") and were assessed on the scale from 1 to 5 (1 "I disagree" to 5 " I agree").

Study staff members assessed the feasibility of HIVST within 24 to 72 hours post-testing by reviewing the documentation of the self-testing process. Study staff recorded the used or unused kits received from the participants. They also recorded the participants' self-test results, as recorded in the interpretation of results form, and compared with the results displayed on the self-test kit. All discrepancies in the interpretation of the self-test results were discussed between the PI and the participant and corrected. In case of invalid self-test results, the PI offered another self-test kit to the participant to test under supervision.

7.4.4 Fidelity of implementation

Fidelity of implementation focused on adherence (i.e. extent of intervention implementation as planned), recruitment of participants (i.e. procedures used to approach participants), dose-delivered (i.e. completed sessions), dose received (i.e. the extent of participants' exposure to the intervention) and reach (i.e. participants' participation rate).

Adherence was assessed by direct observation of PEs at random sequences by an independent observer using a pre-defined index. Adherence was scored from 0 to 2 on 19 aspects of intervention content (range score was 0-38). A score of 0 indicated that the aspect was not implemented, a score of 1 indicated that the aspect was partially implemented and a score of 2 indicated that the aspect was completely implemented. The 19 aspects of the intervention content were grouped into 5 categories as follows: (a) Perceived barriers/facilitators for HIVST uptake (b) myths around HIVST use (c) self-confidence towards HIVST uptake (d) positive or negative consequences of HIVST uptake and (e) skills of using Oral Quick HIVST test kits. PEs' performance on session facilitation was assessed by direct observation at a random sequence by an independent observer. Their performance was scored from 0 to 2 on 9 aspects of session facilitation (range score was 0 18)

A score of 0 indicated that the aspect was not implemented, a score of 1 indicated that aspect was partially implemented and a score of 2 indicated that the aspect was completely implemented.

The 9 aspects of session facilitation were (a) building a friendly relationship with participants, (b) presentation of session objectives, (c) building on participants' experiences,(d) providing reassurance to participants, (e) eliciting and answering questions, (f) listening carefully, (g) checking to understand, (h) eliciting feedback from participants and (i) providing a clear conclusion of the sessions. Recruitment was assessed by the rate of response to invitations delivered to eligible participants. Attendance, length of sessions and retention were recorded by the PEs following each session.

7.4.5 HIVST uptake

Asking participants if they had tested for HIV using HIVST at the 3 months follow-up period assessed HIVST uptake. HIVST uptake was rated using a binary YES/NO response format.

7.4.6 Prevalence of new HIV–positive diagnosis

Prevalence of new HIV-positive diagnosis was the proportion of participants offered HIV testing that were diagnosed HIV positive.

We assessed the number of new HIV–positives by asking all participants who had accepted HIVST to categorize their test results at 3-month follow-up. The outcome options were coded 0=test not working; 1=may have HIV; 2=does not have HIV.

7.4.7 Linkage to HIV prevention

Linkage to HIV prevention was the proportion of individuals with negative test results who sought HIV– prevention services (e.g. voluntary medical male circumcision, condoms, contraception, etc.) within 3 months of being offered the HIVST kits out of all HIV–negative participants.

7.4.8 Linkage to HIV care and treatment

Linkage to HIV care and treatment was the proportion of individuals with positive test results who went for a confirmatory HIV test within 3 months of being offered the HIVST kits and who were initiated to ARV treatment. We assessed linkage to HIV care and treatment by asking participants who reported HIV positive results whether they had sought medical care for confirmatory HIV tests and initiated ARV treatments and reviewed HIV care and treatment clinic records.

7.4.9 Knowledge of HIV testing and HIVST

Knowledge of HIV testing and HIVST was assessed by asking all participants at baseline about whether they knew a place to test for HIV, previous HIV testing history, experiences of using HIVST and whether they knew someone who had ever used HIVST.

7.4.10 Integrated Behavior Model constructs

The before and after changes of the IBM constructs were assessed at 1-month and 3-month follow-up using a pre and post-test semi-structured questionnaire. Participants rated their perceived norms, perceived control and self-efficacy for HIV testing. Table 7.1 below shows knowledge of HIV testing and HIVST and IBM constructs variables and response options measured at both baseline and follow-up survey.

Ā

able 7.1. Knowledge of HIV testing and HIVST and IBM construct variables				
ariable	No. of items	Sample Questions	Scoring	Alpha
nowledge of HIV testing and HIVST				
nows the place to get sted for HIV	NA	Do you know of a place where people go to get the HIV test?	d	
ver been tested for HIV	NA	Have you ever been tested for HIV?	a	
ver used HIVST	NA	Have you ever tested yourself for HIV using a self-test kit?	a	
nows someone who has 'er self-tested	NA	Do you know of someone who has ever tested him/herself using a self-test kit?	a	
3M constructs variables				
junctive norms	8	Most of my friends approve that I should participate in HIV-testing.	b	0.87
escriptive norms	4	Most of my friends think of participating in HIV-testing.	b	0.81
erceived control	7	If I have been drinking alcohol or abusing substances before or while having sex, participating in HIV-testing will be…	b	0.70
elf-efficacy	10	How confident are you that you could participate in HIV-testing?	c	0.78

No'(0), 'Yes'(1)
Scale from 'strongly disagree'(1) to 'strongly agree'(5)
Scale from 'extremely unconfident'(1) to 'extremely confident'(5)

7.5 Procedures

7.5.1 Peer-educators

Before the study initiation, FBWs (n=5) and MCPs (n=5) who were identified by their peers were recruited and trained as peer educators (PEs) by the author **(Chapter Six).** Research assistants visited established bars and through porters' associations within the study setting to collect the names of potential PEs. All PEs were 18 years of age or older and were hired based on their willingness to participate for the duration of the study. After attending a 2 full days of training sessions, PEs visited their peers through their respective social networks. During the visit, PEs informed their peers about the benefits of HIV testing and HIV self-testing in particular to create awareness about HIVST. At the end of the sensitization, PEs offered invitation cards to interested individuals and referred them to the study office within the study settings for eligibility assessment and enrolment. After enrolment, eligible participants were referred to the PEs to schedule attendance at the first intervention sessions.

7.5.2 Baseline survey

A semi-structured paper-based questionnaire for the baseline survey (Appendix H) was distributed to eligible participants between January and March 2018. The Swahili-based questionnaires incorporated four belief-based IBM constructs (i.e. injunctive norm, descriptive norm, perceived control and self-efficacy) because these are most conducive to change (Kasprzyk and Montano 2007). The eligibility criteria for participation were that participants must be over 18 years of age, who have not tested for HIV in the past three months before the date of recruitment, or who are unaware of their HIV status. Four trained research assistants (RAs) explained the purpose and objectives of the study and if participants were eligible and willing, the RAs gained informed consent. RAs conducted the survey, and completion of the questionnaires took an average of 45 minutes. The survey was conducted in a quiet place at the study offices to ensure privacy and confidentiality.

A pilot test was conducted before the baseline survey to assess the validity of the questionnaires. The questionnaire was piloted to a convenient sample of 10 (5 males; 5 females) clients attending a stand-alone VCT centre within the study setting for clarity of language, questions, internal consistency and competency of the four trained RAs. Minor adjustments (i.e. wording, the sequence of questions and coding) were done accordingly.

7.5.3 The IBM behaviour change intervention

The IBM behaviour change intervention -*Jitambue* (the Swahili word for Know your Self) was a multi-component intervention that was based on the Integrated Behavior Model (IBM) (Baranowski et al., 2002, Bandura 2006) and Diffusion of Innovation Theory (DIT) (Oldenburg and Glanz 2008), for implementation of health-related–services (Mavedzenge et al., 2011, WHO 2013, WHO 2014). Findings from systematic reviews **(Chapters Three & Four)** and the formative study with key informants, FBWs and MCPs also informed the development of the IBM behaviour change intervention **(Chapter Five).** The development of the manual-based IBM behaviour change intervention is described in full in **Chapter Six**.

Reporting of the BCI and results followed the Template for Intervention Description and Replication (TIDieR) checklist and guide (Hoffmann et al., 2014). The BCI comprised of an educational strategy, a video on HIVST and a demonstration and simulation on how to use OraQuick® rapid HIV 1/2 antibody test. The intervention consisted of 2 sessions, was delivered by trained PEs at a research centre within Moshi municipality. The session duration ranged from 45 minutes to 60 minutes. Sessions were one-on-one between the PE and participant using motivational interviewing were conducted.

In session one (duration = 60 minutes), the PE presented: (a) information about routes of transmission of HIV to alleviate HIV related misconceptions, and (b) barriers to and facilitators for HIV testing. Then, the PE initiated a discussion to engage in conversation with the participant about HIVST, including its accuracy in detecting antibodies against HIV and on how to use the oral-fluid HIVST kits. This also allowed the participant to learn about the HIVST and clarify any misconceptions about self-testing for HIV.

At the end of session one, the PE scheduled an appointment with the participant for session two within one week.

In session two (duration = 45 minutes), the PE introduced the oral-fluid HIVST under the supervision of the PI [BN]. The study used OraQuick® rapid HIV 1/2 antibody test (OraSure Technologies, Bethlehem, PA, USA), a lateral-flow, immuno-chromatographic, second-generation, oral-fluid assay detecting antibodies to HIV-1 and HIV-2.

The OraQuick is fully WHO pre-qualified and uses oral fluid swabs from upper and lower gums that are placed into are a pre-filled tube of reagent for 20 minutes. When used by laypersons in Kenya, the self-test had a sensitivity of 89.7% and specificity of 98.0% (Thirumurthy et al., 2016). The self-test kits with all the necessary components packaged in a pocket-size plastic pouch were procured through a local agent and distributed to participants free of charge.

Since HIVST is not available in Tanzania, participants viewed a professionally developed video to introduce the concept of HIVST.

The video helped to standardize the information provided to participants and limit interviewer-specific discrepancies in the content and quality of instructions provided. In brief, the video featured an adult African man demonstrating how to use an oral-based HIV test (OraQuick Advance HIV-I/2; OraSure Technologies, Bethlehem, PA), with all instructions in Swahili - a local language familiar to participants. Participants were allowed to view the video twice and were allowed to ask any questions for clarification and were subsequently asked to repeat the demonstration by simulation, using a dummy oral HIVST kit.

Also, participants received an instruction sheet with pictorials in Swahili, adapted from a previous HIVST study in Kenya (Appendix I). The user instructions have images of how to interpret the test window for negative, positive and invalid results (Thirumurthy et al., 2016). Since HIVST can only be used for research purposes in Tanzania, the candidate [BN] distributed the HIVST kits to all participants who agreed to test for HIV, at the end of session two.

According to the manufacturer's recommendations for repeat HIV testing, participants were informed to repeat HIV testing 3 months after receiving a negative test result. Participants reporting a preliminary HIV positive result were informed to seek a confirmatory HIV test immediately.

All participants received a large brown envelope to carry their HIVST kits and were asked to return the used or unused kits in person within one to three days (24-72 hours) at the study office. All participants who received the HIVST kits were provided with a mobile phone number to call if they needed help with using the HIV self-test kits or with any other assistance related to the study.

A participant who reported a preliminary HIV positive result received a referral letter to seek confirmatory HIV testing and initiation of ART at any HIV care and treatment centre of their choice within the study setting. All used kits were discarded as per manufacturer's specifications under the supervision of the candidate

7.5.4 Follow-up survey

A semi-structured paper-based questionnaire for the 3 month follow-up survey (Appendix H) was distributed to eligible participants between June and July 2018. At the 3-month follow-up survey, participants were asked to visit study offices located within Moshi municipality. RAs contacted participants by phone (consent was obtained to make such phone calls and had collected contact details of all participants) to make appointments. If in three consecutive calls the RAs failed to contact a participant, participants were declared lost to follow–up. RAs conducted the survey, and completion of the questionnaires took an average of 60 minutes. The survey was conducted in a quiet place at the study offices to ensure privacy and confidentiality. RAs also recorded all changes in HIV–testing intentions or plans and actual testing during the BCI. Reasons for refusal were carefully documented, along with HIVST experiences and unsuccessful follow-ups. Figure 7.2 below provides the process and timelines of the before-after study design.

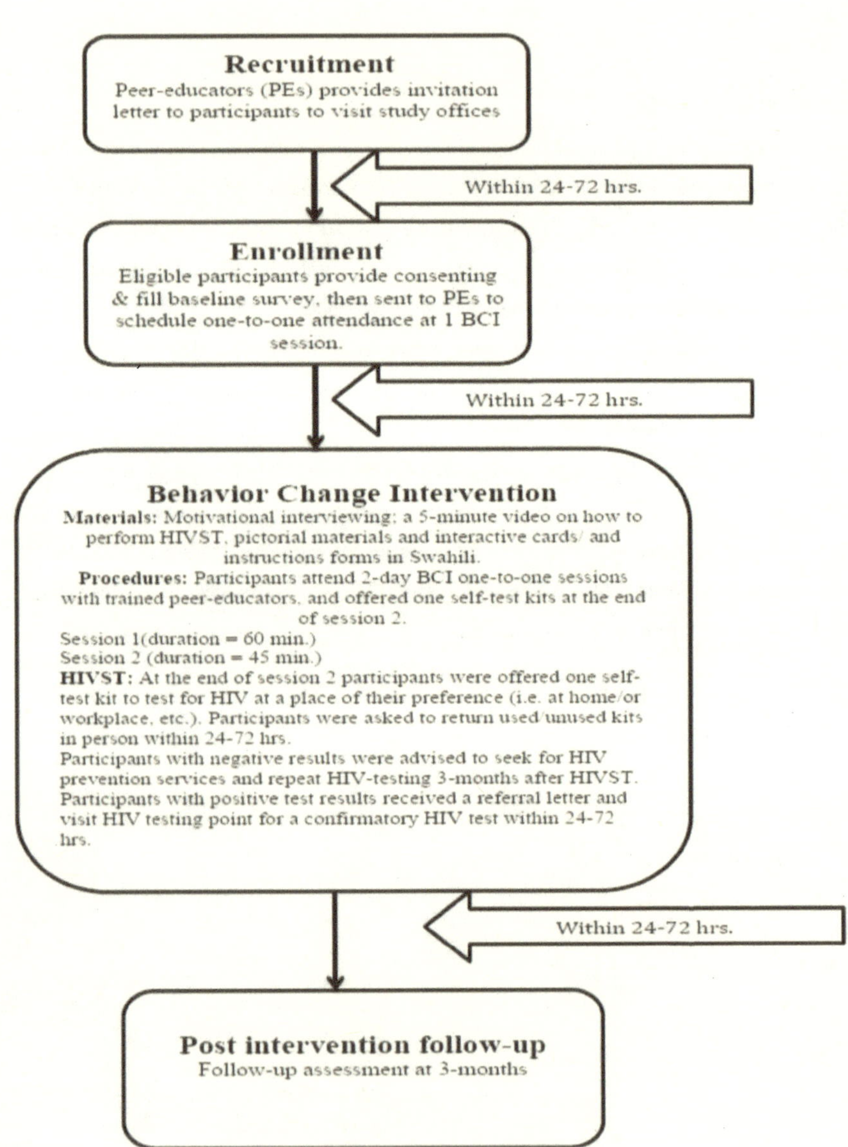

Figure 7.2. The process and timelines of the before-after study design.

7.6 Data analysis

7.6.1 Descriptive analysis

Baseline data were summarized descriptively for participants' demographics, knowledge of HIV testing and HIVST and presented the results using measures of central tendency with their respective measures of dispersion. No comparative statistical analysis was conducted. Adherence and performance scores were presented as mean, standard deviation and percentages.

7.6.2 Bivariate analysis

We performed the internal reliability testing for the items assessing IBM constructs with a cut-off point of Cronbach's alpha coefficient value of 0.6 or higher as satisfactory (Cronbach 1951).

We used a paired sample t-test to calculate mean scores per IBM constructs to assess whether the pre-test and post-test mean differences were statistically different from each other. During the analysis, a reversed Likert scale was used to score the responses with 1 point = neutral; 5 points strongly agree. Eight (8) items assessed the perceived norms (injunctive) construct with a total score ranging from 8 to 40.

A higher score was considered supportive of the BCI. Four (4) items assessed the perceived norms (descriptive) construct with a total score ranging from 4 to 20.

A higher score was considered supportive of the BCI. Seven (7) items assessed the personal agency (perceived control) construct with the total score ranging from 7 to 35. A higher score was considered supportive of the BCI. Ten items assessed the personal agency (self-efficacy) construct with a total score ranging from 10 to 50. A higher score for personal agency (self-efficacy) construct was considered supportive of the BCI.

Ã

7.6.3 Principal component analysis

We conducted the principal component analysis (PCA) to identify the sub-groups of IBM items forming subscales. Before performing PCA, we assessed the suitability of data. The correlation coefficient was set at a cut=off point of .3 or above.

The Kaiser-Meyer-Oklin value- was used to assess sampling adequacy at a cut-off point of .6 (Kaiser 1970, Kaiser 1974), while the Bartlett's test of sphericity supported the factorability of the correlation matrix (Bartlett 1954). Additionally, a Carell's scree test was used and eingen value of over 1.0 for the amount of the total variance explained by a factor (Catell 1966). Further, we performed analysis using Varimax method to minimize the number of variables with high loadings on each factor.

The 32 items of the IBM constructs were subjected to an exploratory PCA. Before conducting PCA, the suitability of the data for factor analysis was assessed. Inspection of the correlation matrix for the IBM constructs revealed the presence of many coefficients of .3 and above. The Kaiser-Meyer-Oklin value was .744, exceeding the cut –off point of .6, and Bartlett's Test of Sphericity was statistically significant (p=0.000). Given the sufficiency of the sample and Kaiser's criterion, we retained all 32 items in the final analysis.

Using a Catell's scree test, 9 components above the breaking point on the scree plots of IBM constructs were retained for further analysis. Further analysis using Varimox method revealed strong loading of the 9 components with eigenvalues exceeding 1, explaining 3.02 per cent, 2.91 per cent, 2.77 per cent, 2.40 per cent, 2.15 per cent, 2.02 per cent, 1.98 per cent, 1.63 per cent and 1.48 per cent. These 9 components explained a total of 73.3 % of the variance.

The 9 items included: injunctive norms = 2 items; descriptive norms = 2 items; and self-efficacy= 5 items. Internal reliability of the items as indicated by Cronbach's alpha coefficients of .767. Table 7.2 below shows the factor loadings after rotation.

Table 7.2. Dimensions of IBM constructs based on Principal Component Analysis			
IBM constructs	Items	Factor loadings [a]	Alpha
Perceived norms (injunctive)	My parents approve that I should participate in HIV testing.	.891	.767
	My spouse approves that I should participate in HIV testing.	.772	
Perceived norms (descriptive)	Most of my other family members think of participating in HIV testing.	.815	
	Most of my friends think of participating in HIV testing.	.790	
Personal agency (self-efficacy)	How confident are you that you could discuss with your spouse/live-in partners on risk reduction after HIV –testing?	.863	
	How confident are you that you could convince your spouse/live-in partner to participate in HIV-testing?	.854	
	How confident are you that you could take HIV testing with your spouse/live-in partner?	.812	
	How confident are you that you could reduce the fear of HIV positive results?	.810	
	How confident are you that you could cope with HIV positive results?	.771	
Factor loadings were extracted using a pattern matrix from varimax rotation			

7.6.4 Qualitative analysis

Qualitative data were analyzed using content analysis (Erlingsson and Brysiewicz 2017). In the first step, two coders listened to the voice recordings and read and re-read transcribed interviews to become familiar and to gain a general understanding of the data. Before analysis, identifying information was removed from the transcripts. While keeping focused on the aim and research question, the transcribed interviews were divided up into smaller parts as the meaning unit. In the second step, the located meaning units were condensed further without losing the essential message of the meaning unit. The aim was to reduce the meaning units that were too large and included many meanings to smaller, manageable data. In the third step, the two coders developed codes that were descriptive labels for the meaning units.

The codes were outlined in a codebook based on the meaning units. The aim was to identify connections between meaning units keeping focused on the data with the minimum interpretation of the content. The two coders combined their codebooks, adjusted and repeated coding, until they reached a consensus of the final codes. In the final step, the codes were sorted into categories aiming to answer the questions: *who, what, when or where*? Codes were compared and appraised to determine which codes seemed to belong together, in order to form categories. Next, themes were generated from a category or categories to answer the questions: *why, how, in what way, or by what means?* The themes expressed underlying meaning and were formed by combining two or more categories. Findings are presented in the results sections with corresponding quotes.

7.7 Results

7.7.1 Acceptability

Out of 183 eligible participants, 179 (97.8 %) accepted the invitation to participate in the BCI. The exit interviews revealed that overall, participants connected well with the peer-educators (PEs). The participants were comfortable interacting with the PEs because they considered them as friends. This was well elaborated by a FBW who said: "*The training was very helpful because our trainers [peer-educators] were just like our friends. We discussed the topics in a very friendly manner because we know each other…*" (FBW aged 28yrs old). Overall, most participants perceived the content and materials of the intervention positively, particularly the video show and demonstration on how to use HIVST. For example, a MCP said: *"All the materials were so helpful, although I liked the video and the demonstration most because I was able to see how to perform the self-testing and also practices on how to use the self-test kits*" (MCP aged 24 yrs. old). In addition, the use of the Swahili language during the training was perceived as very useful: *"…the instructions were in (Ki) Swahili, which was easy to understand very clearly…"* (FBW aged 20 yrs. old).

Participants described the use of picture cards very helpful in session facilitation of the BCI: " *This [self-testing instruction card], is a good one. These pictures are quite self-explanatory like people can look at it and understand what they can do*" (FBW aged 26 yrs. old). Also, participants noted that they were motivated to test for HIV using HIVST after attending the BCI. This is well described in the following narrative by a MCP who stated, "*When I came the first time for the training, I did not know that I would be offered self-testing. After the training I was motivated to use it [HIVST]...*" (MCP aged 27 yrs. old). Discussion on myths towards HIVST, motivational factors and benefits of HIVST increased their knowledge about HIVST, which was perceived as new 'technology' to most participants. As one respondent said: *"Previously, I knew that blood was used to test for HIV and now this new technology of using oral fluids? I wanted to perform HIVST using the self-test kit*!" (MCP aged 22 *yrs. old).*

Participants experienced different levels of emotions while waiting for their HIVST test results. Some participants experienced anxiety, confusion and worry. For example, a FBW gave this narrative: "*I was anxious to know my test result. After collecting the oral fluid from my mouth and putting the brush [collecting device] in the small bottle with fluid [reagent] and waiting for 20 minutes,. I was looking at the display screen and saw a red colouration all over. I was confused...and asked myself ' what is happening now...?'..I continued watching until it started to clear after 10-15 minutes. I was relieved and waited until 20 minutes and I saw my result*" (FBW aged 24 yrs. old). In contrast, some participants were delighted and excited to see their HIV test results, particularly first-time testers: "*I was delighted to see my result after I performed self-testing for the first time in my life. It was a very exciting moment!*" (MCP aged 23 yrs. old).

Finally, participants perceived that the BCI was well planned and interesting: *"It was very interesting to participate in this project [BCI] and be able to test myself for HIV*" (MCP aged 28 yrs. old).

7.7.2 Feasibility

At the end of the sessions, all participants rated their perceptions of intervention sessions and materials. Ratings for the overall intervention sessions ranged from 4.3 to 4.8 (max = 5). Overall rating on materials was between 4.7 and 4.8 (max= 5), as shown in Table 7.3.

Table 7.3. Participants ratings of perceptions on intervention sessions and materials

Items	Mean (SD)
Overall, intervention sessions… [a]	
had a clear structure	4.6(0.6)
taught me something new	4.6(0.6)
were well designed and complete	4.3(0.8)
were understandable	4.7(0.4)
were easy to follow	4.8(0.4)
were arranged in a consistent order	4.6(0.6)
were interesting	4.8(0.4)
were relevant	4.8(0.4)
were useful	4.8(0.4)
were helpful	4.8(0.4)
Overall, the materials presented in the intervention were… [a]	
Understandable	4.8(0.5)
Easy to use	4.8(0.5)
Presented in a consistent order	4.7(0.4)
Interesting	4.8(0.5)
Relevant	4.8(0.5)
Useful	4.7(0.4)
Helpful	4.7(0.4)
[a] Scale from 1 "I disagree" to 5 "I total agree "	

Feasibility of HIVST was assessed within 24 to 72 hrs. post-testing. The majority of participants (98.9%; n= 179) of both FBWs and MCPs recorded their self-testing process correctly. All results were confirmed upon inspection of the used test kits and documentation of interpretation of results. Two participants (1= man; 1= woman) reported invalid test results. The reason for the invalid test results was that the participants did not collect the oral fluid before immersing the collection device in the reagent. Repeat tests were done under supervision and the results were negative. Apart from the two participants who reported invalid test results, the rest of the participants self-tested without supervision.

7.7.3 Fidelity of implementation

The overall mean adherence score was 33.5 (SD 3.2) ranging from 28 to 38 (73 % to 100 %) out of a maximum score of 38. Six out of 10 (60%) of PEs scored above 33.5, indicating moderate adherence to the intervention content. Four of the PEs had scores below 33.5. Intervention components related to skills for HIVST use and perceived barriers/motivators were fully implemented, followed by myths around HIVST use and self - confidence towards HIVST uptake. The least implemented (partially or not implemented) intervention component was related to positive/negative consequences of HIVST uptake (see Table 7. 4).

The overall mean performance score was 15.5 (SD 1.9) ranging from 12 to 18 (66.7 % to 100%) out of a maximum score of 18. Seven of 10 (70%) of PEs scored above 15.5 indicating the high performance of session facilitation. Three of the PEs had scores below 15.5. Sessions facilitation techniques related to eliciting and answering questions and the use of reflective listening were fully implemented, followed by the presentation of session objectives, providing reassurance, reviewing the session objectives, checking to understand, building on participants' experiences and building general rapport. The least implemented (partially or not implemented) facilitation techniques were related to summarizing the sessions. The duration of session 1 varied from 40 to 60 minutes (max= 60 min). The overall mean session duration was 53 min (7.5) and 4 out of 10 (40%) PEs conducted session 1 below 53 min. The duration of session 2 varied from 40 to 45 minutes (max=45 min). The overall mean session duration was 42 min (2.6) and 6 out of 10(60%) PEs conducted session 2 below 42 min (see Table 7.4).

Table 7. 4. Peer educators adherence, performance scores and session duration (N=10)

Items	Mean (SD)
Adherence scores [a]	
Overall mean adherence scores	33.5(3.2)
Perceived barriers/motivators for HIVST	1.8(0.4)
Myths around HIVST	1.7(0.5)
Self-confidence towards HIVST uptake	1.7(0.5)
Positive/negative consequences of HIVST uptake	1.6(0.6)
Skills for HIVST use	1.9(0.3)
Performance scores [a]	
Overall mean performance scores	15.5(1.9)
Build general rapport	1.6(0.7)

Presentation of session objectives	1.8(0.4)
Building on participants experiences	1.7(0.7)
Provide reassurance	1.8(0.4)
Elicit and answer questions	1.9(0.3)
Use reflective listening	1.9(0.3)
Checking to understand	1.7(0.7)
Reviewing the session objectives	1.8(0.4)
Summarizing the sessions	1.3(0.5)
Session duration (in minutes)	
Session 1	53(7.5)
Session 2	42(2.6)
[a] scale from 0 "Not implemented" to 2 "Fully implemented"	

7.7.4 Recruitment rate and retention

Two hundred and twenty-four (n=224) participants (n=110 MCPs; n=114 FBWs) were sampled and invited to participate and 183 (n= 89 MCPs; n= 94 FBWs) consented and were enrolled in the study. This is a recruitment rate of 82.1%. Those who did not meet inclusion criteria included 21 MCPs and 20 FBWs. Three (3) participants declined to participate in the BCI after completing the baseline survey. Reasons mentioned for refusal to participate were lack of time, perceived inaccuracy of HIVST test and fear of positive HIV test results. Out of 89 MCPs, only 1 refused to participate. The remaining 88 MCPs attended both sessions. Out of 94 FBWs, only 2 refused to participate. We considered the proportion of enrolled participants who completed the assessment at 3-months follow-up, with a 60% retention rate being the benchmark for retention. Overall, the retention rate at 3 months follow-up was 99.5% (MCPs = 99%; FBWs = 100%) respectively. Figure 7.3 below

Participant flow chart

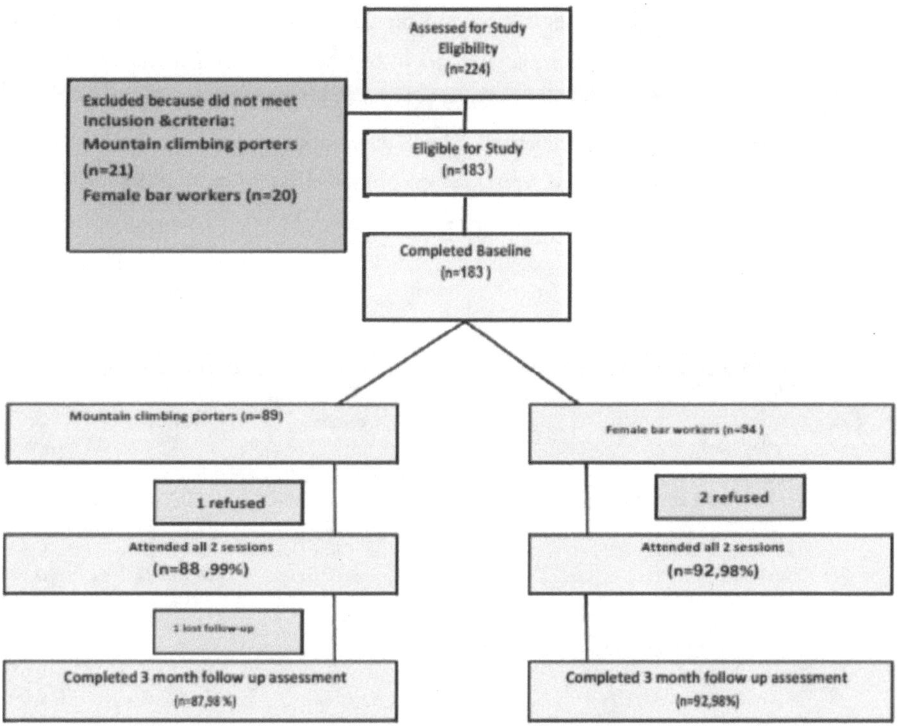

Figure 7. 3. Participant's flow chart

7.7.5 Baseline characteristics of respondents

At baseline, 183 participants (n= 89 MCPs; n= 94 FBWs) participated in this study. The mean age for women was 31 [SD= 7.8]. The mean age for men was 33 [SD= 7.1]. Of the 183 participants, half (51.4%, n= 94) were females.

Almost half, of women (42.6%) and men (47.2%), had primary education, 75.5 % of women and 65.2 % of men were Christians, 52.1% of women and 33.7 % of men were single and 58.5 % of women and 42.7 % of men were living alone.

The majority of both female (98.9%) and male (91%) participants knew a place to test for HIV. The history of those who had previously been tested for HIV differed significantly between women and men (p= 0.001). More women than men (96.8% of women vs. 79.8% of men) self-reported being tested for HIV in their lifetime. More than two-thirds (65. 2 %) of men and 57.8 % of women had tested for HIV within the past 3 months. As expected, very low proportions of both female (8.5%) and male (3.4%) participants had ever used HIVST. Finally, 38.3 % of female participants compared to 29.2% of their male counterparts knew someone who had self-tested for HIV (see Table 7.5).

Table 7.5. Baseline characteristics, knowledge of HIV testing and HIVST of respondents (n=183).

	Females	Males	*p*-value
Variable	N=**94 (51.4%)**	N=**89 (48.6%)**	
Age of participants (Mean ± SD, years)	31±7.8	33±7.1	0.146
Never married	49 (52.1)	30 (33.7)	<0.001
Had primary education	40 (42.6)	42 (47.2)	0.443
Christian	71 (75.5)	58 (65.2)	0.124
Live with husband/wife	18 (19.1)	37 (41.6)	0.001
Living alone	55(58.5)	38(42.7)	0.001
Knowledge of HIV testing and HIVST			
Knows the place to get tested for HIV	93(98.9)	81(91)	0.013
Ever been tested for HIV	91 (96.8)	71 (79.8)	0.001
Recent HIV testing			
Within the past 3 months	54(57.6)	58(65.2)	0.077
Within the past 1 year	40(42.4)	31(34.8%)	0.081
Ever used HIVST	8 (8.5)	3 (3.4)	0.144
Knows someone who has ever self-tested	36(38.3)	26(29.2)	0.194
Use of Family planning (for women only)	55(58.5)	N/A	N/A
Male circumcision	N/A	89(100%)	N/A

7.7.6 HIVST uptake

Of the 183 participants recruited in the study, the majority (97.8%, n=179) participated in the BCI and tested for HIV using the OraQuick HIVST kits. Of the 179 participants, 51.4 % (n=92) were women, while 48.6 % (n= 87) were men and 21 (11.7 %) had never tested for HIV before. Of the 21 first-time testers, 3(14.3%) were women, while 18 (85.7%) were men.

The time elapsed before performing HIVST was almost similar for women and men; 91.3 % of women and 79.3% of men self-tested the same day they received the self-test kits. Two (1 = male; 1=female) participants (1.1%) reported a reactive test result. The majority (98.9 %) of participants reported HIV negative test results when returning the test kits within three days (24 to 72 hours) after receiving the kits.
At the 3-month follow-up, the two participants with a positive HIVST test result reported they had visited a health facility for a confirmatory HIV testing and initiation of ART within 2 weeks post-self-testing. The PI validated the confirmatory HIV test results by checking the facility records. Furthermore, at the 3-month follow-up, one-third (29.3 %, n= 27/94) of women who reported not using any type of family planning (FP) at baseline, reported that they had visited family planning clinics.

Repeat HIV testing (using conventional HTS), 3 months post-HIVST for those who received negative results, differed between men and women. More men than women reported repeat HIV testing 3 months post HIVST; 66.7 % of men and 43.5 % of women went for repeat HIV testing at a health facility (see Table 7.6).

Table 7. 6. Uptake of HIVST (N= 179)

	Females	**Males**	***p*-value**
Variable	N=**94 (51.4%)**	N=**89 (48.6%)**	
Participated in HIVST intervention: (n=183)			
Yes	92(97.9)	87(97.8)	0.956
No	2(2.1)	2(2.2)	
The time before performing HIVST: (n=179)			
Same day	84(91.3)	69(79.3)	0.059
24 hours	5(5.4)	16(18.4)	
More than 24 hours	3(3.3)	2(2.3)	
HIV self-test results: (n= 179)			
Reactive	1(1.1)	1(1.1)	0.818
Negative	91(98.9)	86(98.9)	
Interpretation of results: (n=179)			
Correct interpretation	91(98.9)	86(98.9)	0.391
Incorrect interpretation	1(1.1)	1(1.1)	
Type of HIVST: (n=179)			
Supervised	1(1.1)	1(1.1)	0.503
Unsupervised	91(98.9)	86(98.9)	

Action taken after HIVST (n= 179)			
Went for confirmatory test/started ART	1(1.1)	1(1.1)	0.771
Started family planning	27(29.3)	0(0.0)	
Repeat HIV testing after 3 months of HIVST	40(43.5)	58(66.7)	
Done nothing after HIVST	24(26.1)	28(32.2)	

Ā

7.7.7 Comparison of IBM constructs before and after the intervention

Table 7.7 describes the IBM constructs scores before and after the BCI for perceived norms (injunctive and descriptive norms), perceived control and self-efficacy by gender. The pre and post test scores differed significantly on all measures (p= < 0.001). For both male and female participants, there was a significant increase in three of four IBM constructs scores supportive of the BCI.

For male participants, mean score changes were for descriptive norms, perceived control and self-efficacy (increases of 16.6 to 18.4; 22.4 to 23.6; and 39.4 to 42.8 respectively) and not for injunctive norms (decreases of 22.1 to 19.2).

For female participants, the mean score changes were for descriptive norms, perceived control and self-efficacy (increases of 16.5 to 19.2; 19. 2 to 20.0; and 38.8 to 42.8 respectively) and not for injunctive norms (decreases of 21.1 to 19.4). Table 7.7.

Table 7.7. IBM constructs scores before and after intervention by gender (n=179)

IBM constructs	Male			Female		
	Baseline (Mean ± SD)	Follow-up (Mean ± SD)	p-value	Baseline (Mean ± SD)	Follow-up (Mean ± SD)	p-value
Injunctive norms score	22.1± 3.0	19.2± 1.6	<.0001	21.1 ± 3.4	19.4 ± 2.3	<.0001
Descriptive norms score	16.6± 3.1	18.4±2.8	<.0001	16.5 ± 2.3	19.2 ± 2.4	<.0001
Perceived control score	22.4 ±5.7	23.6 ±5.4	<.0001	19.2 ± 4.5	20.0 ± 5.1	.02
Self-efficacy score	39. 4 ± 3.8	42.8 ±3.1	<.0001	38.8 ± 5.1	42.8 ± 5.4	<.0001

7.8 Discussion

This study used a before-after study design aimed at assessing the impact of a theory-based BCI to increase HIVST uptake and linkage to HIV prevention, care, treatment among FBWs and MCPs in Northern Tanzania.

7.8.1 Baseline findings

At baseline, survey participants demonstrated a high level of HIV and AIDS awareness and knowledge, including on HIV testing. The vast majority of participants were aware of HIV and AIDS, routes of HIV transmission, the efficacy of condoms in HIV prevention and antiretroviral therapy (ART). Further, most participants knew places in their vicinity where they could test for HIV. This observation is in line with studies conducted in other settings in Tanzania, which demonstrated a high level of HIV and AIDS awareness and knowledge (THIS 2017, TENGIA-KESSY and LYAMUYA 2018).

However, this observation is contrary to a study among adolescents in rural Mozambique, which observed a limited knowledge of HIV transmission (Hector et al., 2018). Contrary, most participants in this study were unaware of HIVST before the survey. This is not a surprising finding since HIVST is regarded as a 'new' technology for HTS and corroborates similar results from SSA (Mokgatle and Madiba 2017, Conserve et al., 2018a, Conserve et al., 2018b, Hector et al., 2018, Tonen-Wolyec et al., 2018).

7.8.2 Acceptability and feasibility

The present results suggest that BCI is acceptable to FBWs and MCPs and feasible in an urban setting in Northern Tanzania. Most study participants perceived the use of trained peer-educators who were selected among study participants very helpful. This observation may explain the high levels of acceptability reported in the current study. Systematic review evidence suggests that peer-education interventions are associated with high acceptability of HIV prevention, including increasing HIV knowledge, HIV prevention among injection drug uses and condom use (Medley et al., 2009).

The acceptability of peer-education interventions is related to the strong influence that peers have on individual behaviour and the level of trust and comfort with their peers that allows for more open discussions of sensitive topics (Ford et al., 2008, Geibel et al., 2012, Onyango et al., 2016, Chanda et al., 2017, Oldenburg et al., 2017).

Study participants accepted the content, materials and procedures used in the BCI. This was indicated by high ratings from participants' feedback. The helpfulness of specific materials was reported, particularly for the video show. Also, participants appreciated the use of Swahili as the medium for instruction during training. In addition, participants mentioned the use of pictorials was very helpful.

Previous studies have reported the use of a clear, well-understood language and the use of visual aids and pictorial images help in increased identification with the information and messaging (Ng et al., 2012, Figueroa et al., 2015, Ortblad et al., 2018).

Discussion on misconceptions about HIVST helped participants to regulate their negative feelings about HIVST. This helped to provide insight into the perception of HIVST as a new 'technology'. From the theoretical perspective, regulating negative emotions related to behaviour is fundamental in the behaviour change process (Tavender et al., 2015).

The feasibility of HIVST was high, with the majority of participants correctly documenting their self-testing process. Additionally, two invalid test results were documented in this study. This observation is in line with findings from other settings, where invalid test results are a common problem of HIVST with the variability of rates between settings and populations (Ng et al., 2012, Kurth et al., 2016, Hector et al., 2018).

In the current study, the reason for the invalid test result was related to errors in sample collection, which has been documented in other studies as a reason for invalid HIVST results (Peck et al., 2014, Kurth et al., 2016).

This observation suggests the need for adequate supportive materials and resources accompanying the distribution of self-test kits, which will improve participants' skills and confidence in the usage of the kits (Zanolini et al., 2017).

Ā

7.8.3 Fidelity of implementation

Evidence for the fidelity of implementation varied for adherence and performance scores of trained PEs. The study findings indicate a moderate level of fidelity of adherence to the specified BCTs and a high level of fidelity of performance of session facilitation. These findings suggest that trained PEs implemented most BCTs and session facilitation skills fully. Other contributing factors for the fidelity of implementation include the optimal length of training sessions and successful recruitment and retention rates in this study. Ā

7.8.4 HIVST uptake

The study findings demonstrated high HIVST uptake among targeted populations in this setting. This finding concurs with studies on the uptake of HIVST from different settings (Lee et al., 2007, Krause et al., 2013, Pai et al., 2013, Chipungu et al., 2017, Figueroa et al., 2018). This observation could be explained by the fact that participants were offered HIV using the OraQuick HIVST kits.

Existing evidence from other studies from SSA suggest that the majority of participants preferred oral HIVST compared to blood-based test because it is easy to use and less invasive because of the absence of a finger prick (Njau et al., 2016, Sarkar et al., 2016, Mugo et al., 2017).

The HIV positive results reported by participants from the HIVST was low and does not support the idea that MCPs and FBWs are at particularly high risk for HIV infection. An explanation could be that no eligible participants who knew they were HIV positive were included in this study. The rationale of excluding known HIV positive participants was to avoid overestimation of new HIV positive diagnosis (Sharma et al., 2015, Johnson et al., 2017). An alternative explanation could be that those MCPs and FBWs who are at higher risk are even harder to reach.

Our study was able to reach people who had never tested for HIV before and concurs with findings, which reported that HIVST could identify and reach first-time testers because it provides an opportunity for individuals to test for HIV. The first-time tester in this study was excited to test for HIV for the first time in his lifetime by doing self-testing for HIV.

These findings indicate the potential of HIVST to reach first-time testers and may be beneficial for hard-to-reach populations who have never tested for HIV before (Krause et al., 2013, Suthar et al., 2013, Hatzold et al., 2019).

In this study, linkage to care and ART initiation following a positive HIVST was reported. At the 3-month follow-up, the two participants who received HIV positive results reported visiting a health facility for confirmatory HIV testing and initiated ART within 2 weeks post-HIV self-test. This result should be interpreted with caution because the current study lacks baseline data on the linkage of HIV care and treatment for comparison among the target population in the study setting.

Participants who reported a negative HIV self-test were offered information about HIV prevention services including Voluntary Medical Male Circumcision (VMMC) and family planning. At baseline, all-male participants self-reported they had undergone VMMC, which was not a surprising finding because of an ongoing campaign in Tanzania to promote VMMC since 2010 (Mahler et al., 2011).

Almost one-third of female participants who did not use any type of family planning at baseline reported at the 3-month follow-up visiting a family planning clinic after attending the BCI. Provision of preventive materials and support by peer-educators may have facilitated family planning seeking behaviour of women in this study setting.

Our study findings reported that more than half of the participants went to a health facility for a repeat HIV test 3 –months after receiving a negative HIV self-test.

This is in line with Tanzania's national HIV testing algorithm (United Republic of Tanzania and Ministry of Health and Social Welfare National AIDS Control Programme (NACP) 2012) and the finding suggests that an HIVST intervention such as the current study may encourage repeat HIV testing in this hard-to-reach population.

Lastly, all participants in the current study found that the oral HIVST kits were very easy to use, in the privacy of their place and convenient time. This observation concurs with findings reported from HIVST studies conducted in other settings. (Njau et al., 2016, Sarkar et al., 2016, Mugo et al., 2017) In this study, the few participants who refused to participate in the intervention mentioned perceived inaccuracy of the oral HIVST kits, fear of a positive test result and inability to perform HIVST alone as reasons for their refusal to participate. Similar concerns have been reported from HIVST studies and underline the importance of addressing impediments for HIVST uptake (Choko et al., 2017, Indravudh et al., 2017, Knight et al., 2017, Mugo et al., 2017, Indravudh et al., 2018).ÂÂ

7.8.5 Before and after changes of the IBM constructs

The study findings indicated increased scores of descriptive norms, perceived control and self-efficacy for female and male participants, with a statistically significant difference between pre-test and post-test. This coincides with other multiple intervention clinics and community-based studies and meta-analyses, showing self-efficacy is an important construct that affects the likelihood of performing the intended behaviour (Kasprzyk et al., 1998, Baranowski et al., 2002, Kasprzyk and Montano 2007, Scott-Sheldon et al., 2011, Montaño et al., 2014). This observation suggests the importance of a sense of confidence over-social-psychological barriers to use HIVST. In the HIV testing context, self-efficacy might have a significant influence on the way the target population confronts HIV/AIDS-related stressors.

According to IBM, both injunctive and descriptive norms are important constructs of social influence in social identity and might influence the uptake of recommended behaviour such as HIVST (Kasprzyk et al., 1998, Baranowski et al., 2002, Kasprzyk and Montano 2007, Montaño et al., 2014).

However, in this study, the injunctive norms scores decreased for both male and female participants post-test, suggesting that the intervention failed to change the injunctive norms compared to the remaining four IBM constructs.

According to Baranowski (2002), the injunctive norm is an individual's belief about the extent to which other people who are important to them think they should or should not perform a particular behaviour (Baranowski et al., 2002). However, given the nature of HIVST, which provides autonomy and perceived self-control of the individual's ownership of testing for HIV; participants might find injunctive norms as less significant in their decision-making process. An alternative explanation for this observation could be due to methodological limitations during the design of the intervention. We speculate that maybe the key normative beliefs included in the intervention were insufficient to bring about the anticipated change. From a theoretical perspective, Fishbein and Cappella (Fishbein and Cappella 2006), argue that not all beliefs are equally susceptible to direct change and may also vary across population subgroups, which could be an alternative explanation. Future BCI using the IBM constructs should consider how best to change injunctive norms.

7.8.6 Limitations

Several limitations need to be considered when interpreting the findings of this study. First, we used a before-after study design instead of a clinical trial to evaluate the impact of the BCI.

Potential limitations of this study design include lack of a comparison or control group, inability to establish a causal-effect relationship between exposure and the outcome, inability to take into account temporal changes independent of the intervention and regression to mean. Despite these potential limitations, the study design was found feasible for the evaluation of the BCI due to low cost, convenience and simplicity compared to an RCT.

Second, the findings of this study may have limited generalizability to the general population of young people in Tanzania.

Third, the results are based on participants' self-reports. In responding to sensitive topics such as HIV testing, participants may have over-reported or under-reported their HIV testing behaviours. This may introduce social desirability bias, which is very common with self-reporting. Another limitation is that participants' report of the use of the HIVST kits may be subject to social desirability bias.

For example, participants may want to report that they used the HIVST kit when they did not. To reduce these bias, participants were asked to return the HIVST kits, either used or unused, within three days (24 to 72 hours) after receiving the kits, in order to ascertain the actual use of the HIVST kits. Moreover, this study was limited to using oral-fluid based self-tests kits. Further studies are warranted to also understand preferences for whole blood-based self-tests in this population and setting.

7.9 Conclusion

The present findings suggest the BCI was well acceptable among FBWs and MCPs and feasible in an urban setting in northern Tanzania. The BCI was implemented with moderate to high levels of fidelity by trained PEs. Additionally, the study findings make an important contribution to the literature on the potential for a theory-based BCI to increase HIVST uptake and linkage to HIV prevention, treatment and care.

References

Ahmed, S., Delaney, K., Villalba-Diebold, P., Aliyu, G., Constantine, N., Ememabelem, M. . . . Charurat, M. (2013). HIV counselling and testing and access-to-care needs of populations most-at-risk for HIV in Nigeria. *AIDS Care, 25*(1), 85-94. Doi:10.1080/09540121.2012.686597

Ao, T. T., Sam, N. E., Masenga, E. J., Seage, G. R., & Kapiga, S. H. (2006). Human Immunodeficiency Virus Type 1 among Bar and Hotel Workers in Northern Tanzania: The Role of Alcohol, Sexual Behaviour and Herpes Simplex Virus Type 2. *Sexually Transmitted Diseases, 33*(3), 163-169. Doi:10.1097/01.olq.0000187204.57006.b3

Asiimwe, S., Oloya, J., Song, X., & Whalen, C. C. (2014). Accuracy of un-supervised versus provider-supervised self-administered HIV testing in Uganda: A randomized implementation trial. *AIDS Behaviour, 18*(12), 2477-2484. Doi: 10.1007/s10461-014-0765-4

Bandura, A. (2006). GUIDE FOR CONSTRUCTING SELF-EFFICACY SCALES, In A. Bandura (Ed.), *Self-Efficacy Beliefs of Adolescents* (pp. 307-337): Information Age Publishing.

Baranowski, T., Perry, C., & Parcel, G. (2002). How individuals, environments and health behavior interact: Social Cognitive Theory. In K. Glanz, B. Rimer & F. M. Lewis (Eds.), Health Behaviour and Health Education: Theory, research and practice (3rd ed., pp. 165-184). San Francisco: Jossey-Bass.

Bartlett, M. S. (1954). A note on the multiplying factors for various chi-square approximations. *J Roy*

Brown, B., Folayan, M. O., Imosili, A., Durueke, F., & Amuamuziam, A. (2015). HIV self-testing in Nigeria: Public opinions and perspectives. *Global public health, 10*(3), 354-365. Retrieved from http://www.tandfonline.com/Doi/pdf/10.1080/17441692.2014.947303

Cambiano, V., Ford, D., Mabugu, T., Napierala Mavedzenge, S., Miners, A., Mugurungi, O. . . . Phillips, A. (2015). Assessment of the Potential Impact and Cost-effectiveness of Self-Testing for HIV in Low-Income Countries. *J Infect Dis, 212*(4), 570-577. Doi:10.1093/infdis/jiv040

Cattell, R. B. (1966). The scree test for numbers of factors. *Multivariate Behaviour Research, 1*, 245-276.

Chanda, M. M., Ortblad, K. F., Mwale, M., Chongo, S., Kanchele, C., Kamungoma, N. . . . Oldenburg, C. E. (2017). HIV self-testing among female sex workers in Zambia: A cluster randomized controlled trial. *PLoS Medicine, 14*(11), e1002442. Doi:10.1371/journal.pmed.1002442

Chipungu, J., Bosomprah, S., Zanolini, A., Thimurthy, H., Chilengi, R., Sharma, A., & Holmes, C. B. (2017). Understanding linkage to care with an HIV self-test approach in Lusaka, Zambia - A mixed-method approach. *PLoS ONE, 12*(11), e0187998. Doi:10.1371/journal.pone.0187998

Choko, A. T., Desmond, N., Webb, E. L., Chavula, K., Napierala-Mavedzenge, S., Gaydos, C. A. . . . Corbett, E. L. (2011). The uptake and accuracy of oral kits for HIV self-testing in high HIV prevalence setting a cross-sectional feasibility study in Blantyre, Malawi. *PLoS Medicine, 8*(Critical Appraisal Skills Programme 2010), e1001102. Doi:10.1371/journal.pmed.1001102

Choko, A. T., Fielding, K., Stallard, N., Maheswaran, H., Lepine, A., Desmond, N. . . . Corbett, E. L. (2017). Investigating interventions to increase uptake of HIV testing and linkage into care or prevention for male partners of pregnant women in antenatal clinics in Blantyre, Malawi: study protocol for a cluster-randomized trial. *Trials, 18*(1), 349. Doi: 10.1186/s13063-017-2093-2

Choko, A. T., Kumwenda, M. K., Johnson, C. C., Sakala, D. W., Chikalipo, M. C., Fielding, K., . . . Corbett, E. L. (2017). Acceptability of woman-delivered HIV self-testing to the male partner and additional interventions: a qualitative study of antenatal care participants in Malawi. *Journal of the International Aids Society, 20*(1), 1-10. Doi:10.7448/IAS.20.1.21610

Choko, A. T., MacPherson, P., Webb, E. L., Willey, B. A., Feasy, H., Sambakunsi, R. . . . Corbett, E. L. (2015). Uptake, Accuracy, Safety and Linkage into Care over Two Years of Promoting Annual Self-Testing for HIV in Blantyre, Malawi: A Community-Based Prospective Study. *PLoS Medicine, 12*(Effective Practice and Organisation of Care 2009), e1001873. Doi:10.1371/journal.pmed.1001873

Conserve, D., Kajula, L., Yamanis, T., & Maman, S. (2016). Formative Research to Develop Human Immunodeficiency Virus (HIV) Self-Testing Intervention among Networks of Men in Dar es Salaam, Tanzania: A Mixed Methods Approach. *Open Forum Infectious Diseases, Volume 3, Issue suppl_1, 3,* (1,), 518, Retrieved from https://Doi.org/10.1093/ofid/ofw172.381

Conserve, D. F., Alemu, D., Yamanis, T., Maman, S., & Kajula, L. (2018a). "He Told Me to Check My Health": A Qualitative Exploration of Social Network Influence on Men's HIV Testing Behaviour and HIV Self-Testing Willingness in Tanzania. *American Journal of Men's Health.*

Conserve, D. F., Muessig, K. E., Maboko, L. L., Shirima, S., Kilonzo, M. N., Maman, S., & Kajula, L. (2018b). Mate Yako Afya Yako: Formative research to develop the Tanzania HIV self-testing education and promotion (Tanzania STEP) project for men. *PLoS ONE.* Doi:10.1371/journal.pone.0202521

Critical Appraisal Skills Programme 2010. (Critical Appraisal Skills Programme 2010). Critical Appraisal Skills Programme (CASP). 10 questions to help you make sense of qualitative research. England: Critical Appraisals Skills Programme 2010. Retrieved from http://www.casp-uk.net/wp-content/uploads/2011/11/CASP Qualitative Appraisal Checklist 14oct10.pdf.

Cronbach, L. J. (1951). Coefficient alpha and the internal structure of tests. *Psychometrika, 16*, 297-334.

Figueroa, C., Johnson, C., Ford, N., Sands, A., Dalal, S., Meurant, R. . . . Baggaley, R. (2018). Reliability of HIV rapid diagnostic tests for self-testing compared with testing by health-care workers: a systematic review and meta-analysis. *The Lancet HIV*. Doi: 10.1016/s2352-3018(18)30044-4

Fishbein, M., & Cappella, J. N. (2006). The role of theory in developing effective health communications. *Journal of Communication, 56*(S1-S17.), S1-S17. Doi: 10.1111/J.1460-2466.2006.00280.X

Ford, K., Wirawan, D. N., Suastina, W., Reed, B. D., & Muliawan, P. (2008). Evaluation of a peer education programme for female sex workers in Bali, Indonesia. *International Journal of STD AIDS, 11*, 731–733.

Gagnon, M., French, M., & Hebert, Y. (2018). The HIV self-testing debate: where do we stand? *BMC Int Health Hum Rights, 18*(1), 5. Doi: 10.1186/s12914-018-0146-6

Geibel, S., King'ola, N., Temmerman, M., & Luchters, S. (2012). The impact of peer outreach on HIV knowledge and prevention behaviours of male sex workers in Mombasa, Kenya. *Sexually Transmitted Infections, 88*, 357–362. Retrieved from https://sti.bmj.com/content/88/5/357.long

Hatzold, K., Gudukeya, S., Mutseta, M. N., Chilongosi, R., Nalubamba, M., Nkhoma, C. . . . Corbett, E. L. (2019). HIV self-testing: breaking the barriers to uptake of testing among men and adolescents in sub-Saharan Africa, experiences from STAR demonstration projects in Malawi, Zambia and Zimbabwe. *J Int AIDS Soc, 22 Suppl 1*, e25244. Doi:10.1002/jia2.25244.

Hector, J., Davies, M. A., Dekker-Boersema, J., Aly, M. M., Abdalad, C. C. A., Langa, E. B. R. . . . Jefferys, L. F. (2018). Acceptability and performance of a directly assisted oral HIV self-testing intervention in adolescents in rural Mozambique. *PLoS ONE, 13*(4), e0195391. Doi:10.1371/journal.pone.0195391

Hoffmann, T. C., Glasziou, P. P., Boutron, I., Milne, R., Perera, R., Moher, D. . . . Michie, S. (2014). Better reporting of interventions: template for intervention description and replication (TIDieR) checklist and guide. *BMJ, 348*, g1687. doi:10.1136/bmj.g1687

Indravudh, P. P., Choko, A. T., & Corbett, E. L. (2018). Scaling up HIV self-testing in sub-Saharan Africa: a review of technology, policy and evidence. *Current Opinion Infectious Diseases, 31*(1), 14-24. Doi:10.1097/QCO.0000000000000426

Indravudh, P. P., Sibanda, E. L., d'Elbee, M., Kumwenda, M. K., Ringwald, B., Maringwa, G. . . . Taegtmeyer, M. (2017). 'I will choose when to test, where I want to test': investigating young people's preferences for HIV self-testing in Malawi and Zimbabwe. *AIDS, 31 Suppl 3*, S203-S212. doi:10.1097/QAD.0000000000001516

Jennings, L., Conserve, D. F., Merrill, J., Kajula, L., Iwelunmor, J., Linnemayr, S., & Maman, S. (2017). Perceived Cost Advantages and Disadvantages of Purchasing HIV Self- Testing Kits among Urban Tanzanian Men: An Inductive Content Analysis. *Journal of AIDS & Clinical Research, 08*(08). Doi:10.4172/2155-6113.1000725

Kaiser, H. (1970). A Second-generation Little Jiffy. *Psychometrika, 35*, 401-415.

Kaiser, H. (1974). An index of factorial simplicity. *Psychometrika, 39*, 31-36.

Kalibala, S., Tun, W., Cherutich, P., Nganga, A., Oweya, E., & Oluoch, P. (2014). Factors associated with acceptability of HIV self-testing among health care workers in Kenya. *AIDS Behaviour, 18 Suppl 4*, S405-414. Doi: 10.1007/s10461-014-0830-z.

Kapiga, S. H., Sam, N. E., Shao, J. F., Renjifo, B., Massenga, E. J., Kiwelu, I. E., & Essex, M. (2002). HIV-1 Epidemic among Female Bar Workers and Hotel Workers in Northern Tanzania: Risk Factors and Opportunities for Prevention. *Journal of Acquired Immune Deficiency Syndromes, 29(4)*, 409-417.

Kasprzyk, D., Montana, D. E., & Fishbein, M. (1998). Application of an Integrated Behavior Model to Predict Condom Use: A prospective study among High HIV Risk Groups. *Journal of Applied Social Psychology, 28*(17), 1557-1583.

Kasprzyk, D., & Montano, D. (2007). Application of an integrated behavior model to understand HIV prevention behaviour of high-risk men in rural Zimbabwe.

Knight, L., Makusha, T., Lim, J., Peck, R., Taegtmeyer, M., & van Rooyen, H. (2017). "I think it is right": a qualitative exploration of the acceptability and desired future use of oral swab and finger-prick HIV self-tests by lay users in KwaZulu-Natal, South Africa. *BMC Research Notes, 10*(1), 486. Doi: 10.1186/s13104-017-2810-7

Krause, J., Subklew-Sehume, F., Kenyon, C., & Colebunders, R. (2013). Acceptability of HIV self-testing: a systematic literature review. *BMC Public Health, 13* :(735.), 1-19.

Kumwenda, M., Munthali, A., Phiri, M., Mwale, D., Guttenberg, T., MacPherson, E. . . . Desmond, N. (2014). Factors shaping initial decision-making to self-test amongst cohabiting couples in urban Blantyre, Malawi. *AIDS Behaviour, 18 Suppl 4*, S396-404. Doi: 10.1007/s10461-014-0817-9

Kurth, A. E., Cleland, C. M., Chhun, N., Sidle, J. E., Were, E., Naanyu, V. . . . Siika, A. M. (2016). Accuracy and Acceptability of Oral Fluid HIV Self-Testing in a General Adult Population in Kenya. *AIDS Behaviour, 20*(4), 870-879. Doi: 10.1007/s10461-015-1213-9

Lee, V. J., Tan, S. C., Earnest, A., Seong, P. S., Tan, H. H., & Leo, Y. S. (2007). User acceptability and feasibility of self-testing with HIV rapid tests. *Journal of Acquired Immune Deficiency Syndromes, 45*(4), 449-453. Doi:10.1097/QAI.0b013e318095a3f3

Lenth, R. (2001). Some Practical Guidelines for Effective Sample Size Determination. *The American Statistician, 55*(3), 187-193. Doi 10.1198/000313001317098149

Lyamuya, J. E., Njau, B., Damian, D. J., & Mtuy, T. (2017). Sociodemographic and Other Characteristics Associated With Behavioural Risk Factors of HIV Infection Among Male Mountain-Climbing Porters in Kilimanjaro Region, Tanzania. *East African Health Research Journal*, 1-8. Retrieved from www.eahealth.org

Mahler, H. R., Kileo, B., Curran, K., Plotkin, M., Adamu, T., Hellar, A. . . . Fimbo, B. (2011). Voluntary Medical Male Circumcision: Matching Demand and Supply with Quality and Efficiency in a High-Volume Campaign in Iringa Region, Tanzania. *PLoS Medicine, 8*(11), 1-8. Doi:10.1371/journal.pmed.1001131

Makusha, T., Knight, L., Taegtmeyer, M., Tulloch, O., Davids, A., Lim, J. . . . van Rooyen, H. (2015). HIV Self-Testing Could "Revolutionize Testing in South Africa, but It Has Got to Be Done Properly": Perceptions of Key Stakeholders. *PLoS ONE, 10*(3), e0122783. Doi:10.1371/journal.pone.0122783

Matovu, J. K. B., Kisa, R., Buregyeya, E., Chemusto, H., Mugerwa, S., Musoke, W. . . . Wanyenze, R. K. (2018). 'If I had not taken it [HIVST kit] home, my husband would not have come to the facility to test for HIV': HIV self-testing perceptions, delivery strategies and post-test experiences among pregnant women and their male partners in Central Uganda. *Global health action, 11*(1), 1503784. Doi:10.1080/16549716.2018.1503784

Mavedzenge, S. N., Baggaley, R., & Corbett, E. L. (2013). A review of self-testing for HIV: research and policy priorities in a new era of HIV prevention. *Clinical Infectious Diseases, 57*(1), 126-138.

Mavedzenge, S. N., Baggaley, R., Lo, Y. R., & Corbett, L. (2011). HIV self-testing among health workers: a review of the literature and discussion of current practices, issues and options for increasing access to HIV testing in Sub-Saharan Africa.

Mokgatle, M. M., & Madiba, S. (2017). High Acceptability of HIV Self-Testing among Technical Vocational Education and Training College Students in Gauteng and North West Province: What Are the Implications for the Scale-Up in South Africa? *PLoS ONE, 12*(1), e0169765. Doi:10.1371/journal.pone.0169765

Montan˜o, D. E., Kasprzyk, D., Hamilton, D. T., Tshimanga, M., & Gorn, G. (2014). Evidence-Based Identification of Key Beliefs Explaining Adult Male Circumcision Motivation in Zimbabwe: Targets for Behaviour Change Messaging. *AIDS Behaviour, 18*, 885–904.

Morfaw, F., Mbuagbaw, L., Thabane, L., Rodrigues, C., Wunderlich, A. P., Nana, P., & Kunda, J. (2013). Male involvement in prevention programs of mother to child transmission of HIV: a systematic review to identify barriers and facilitators. *Syst Rev, 2*, 5. Doi: 10.1186/2046-4053-2-5

Morin, S. F., Khumalo-Sakutukwa, G., Charlebois, E. D., Routh, J., Fritz, K., & Lane, T. (2006).

Removing barriers to knowing HIV status: same-day mobile HIV testing in Zimbabwe.

http://graphics.tx.ovid.com/ovftpdfs/FPDDNCLBABCDJD00/fs047/ovft/live/gv031/00126334/00126334-200602010-00014.pdf.

Mugo, P. M., Micheni, M., Shangala, J., Hussein, M. H., Graham, S. M., Rinke de Wit, T. F., & Sanders, E. J. (2017). Uptake and Acceptability of Oral HIV Self-Testing among Community Pharmacy Clients in Kenya: A Feasibility Study. *PLoS ONE, 12*(1), e0170868. Doi:10.1371/journal.pone.0170868

Mukolo, A., Blevins, M., Victor, B., Paulin, H. N., Vaz, L. M., Sidat, M., & Vergara, A. E. (2013). Community stigma endorsement and voluntary counselling and testing behavior and attitudes among female heads of household in Zambezia Province, Mozambique. *BMC Public Health, 13*, 1155. Doi: 10.1186/1471-2458-13-1155.

Musheke, M., Ntalasha, H., Gari, S., McKenzie, O., Bond, V., Martin-Hilber, A., & Merten, S. (2013). A systematic review of qualitative findings on factors enabling and deterring uptake of HIV testing in Sub-Saharan Africa. *BMC Public Health, 13*, 220. Doi: 10.1186/1471-2458-13-220

Negin, J., Wariero, J., Mutuo, P., Jan, S., & Pronyk, P. (Effective Practice and Organisation of Care 2009). Feasibility, acceptability and cost of home-based HIV testing in rural Kenya. *Tropical Medicine and International Health, 14*(8), 849-855. Doi:10.1111/j.1365-3156.2009.02304.x

Neuman, M., Indravudh, P., Chilongosi, R., d'Elbee, M., Desmond, N., Fielding, K. . . . Corbett, E. L. (2018). The effectiveness and cost-effectiveness of community-based lay distribution of HIV self-tests in increasing uptake of HIV testing among adults in rural Malawi and rural and peri-urban Zambia: protocol for STAR (self-testing for Africa) cluster randomized evaluations. *BMC Public Health, 18*(1), 1234. Doi: 10.1186/s12889-018-6120-3

Ng, O. T., Chow, A. L., Lee, V. J., Chen, M. I. C., Win, M. K., Tan, H. H., . . . Leo, Y. S. (2012). Accuracy and User-Acceptability of HIV Self-Testing Using an Oral fluid-based HIV Rapid Test. *PLoS ONE 7(Effective Practice and Organisation of Care 2009): e45168.* Doi*:10.1371/journal.pone.0045168.*

Njau, B., Damian, D. J., Abdullahi, L., Boulle, A., & Mathews, C. (2016). The effects of HIV self-testing on the uptake of HIV testing and linkage to antiretroviral treatment among adults in Africa: a systematic review protocol. *Systematic Reviews, 5*(1), 1-8. Doi: 10.1186/s13643-016-0230-8

Njau, B., Ostermann, J., Brown, D., Muhlbacher, A., Reddy, E., & Thielman, N. (2014). HIV testing preferences in Tanzania: a qualitative exploration of the importance of confidentiality, accessibility and quality of service. *BMC Public Health, 14*, 838. Doi: 10.1186/1471-2458-14-838

Njau, B., Watt, M. H., Ostermann, J., Manongi, R., & Sikkema, K. J. (2012). Perceived acceptability of home-based couples voluntary HIV counselling and testing in Northern Tanzania. *AIDS Care, 24*(4), 413-419. Doi:10.1080/09540121.2011.608796

Oldenburg, B., & Glanz, K. (2008). Diffusion of Innovations. In K. In Glanz, F. M. Lewis, & K. Viswanath (Eds.), *Health Behaviour and Health Education: Theories, research and practice*. (Vol. 4th Edition, pp. 313-333). San Fransisco: Jossey-Bass.

Oldenburg, C. E., Ortblad, K. F., Chanda, M. M., Mwanda, K., Nicodemus, W., Sikaundi, R. . . . Barnighausen, T. (2017). Zambian Peer Educators for HIV Self-Testing (ZEST) study: rationale and design of a cluster-randomized trial of HIV self-testing among female sex workers in Zambia. *BMJ Open, 7*(4), e014780. Doi: 10.1136/bmjopen-2016-014780

Onyango, M. A., Adu-Sarkodie, Y., Agyarko-Poku, T., Asafo, M. K., Sylvester, J., Wondergem, P. . . . Beard, J. (2016). "It's all about making a life": poverty, HIV, violence and other vulnerabilities faced by young female sex workers in Kumasi, Ghana. *Journal of AIDS, 68*, S131–137.

Ostermann J, Whetten K, Reddy E, Pence B, Weinhold A, Itemba D . . . Team, C. R. (2014). Treatment retention and care transitions during and after the scale-up of HIV care and treatment in Northern Tanzania. *AIDS Care. 2014; 26(11):1352-8.* Doi:10.1080/09540121.2014.882493.

Ostermann, J., Njau, B., Brown, D. S., Muhlbacher, A., & Thielman, N. (2014). Heterogeneous HIV testing preferences in an urban setting in Tanzania: results from a discrete choice experiment.

Ostermann, J., Njau, B., Mtuy, T., Brown, D. S., Muhlbacher, A., & Thielman, N. (2015). One size does not fit all: HIV testing preferences differ among high-risk groups in Northern Tanzania. *AIDS Care, 27*(5), 595-603. Doi:10.1080/09540121.2014.998612.

Pai, N. P., Sharma, J., Shivkumar, S., Pillay, S., Vadnais, C., Joseph, L. . . . Peeling, R. W. (2013). Supervised and Unsupervised Self-Testing for HIV in High- and Low-Risk Populations: A Systematic Review. *PLoS Medicine, 10(4):* e1001414.

Pant Pai, N., Behlim, T., Abrahams, L., Vadnais, C., Shivkumar, S., Pillay, S. . . . Dheda, K. (2013). Will an Unsupervised Self-Testing Strategy for HIV Work in Health Care Workers of South Africa? A Cross-Sectional Pilot Feasibility Study. *PLoS ONE, 8*(11). Doi:10.1371/journal.pone.0079772

Peaty, D. (Critical Appraisal Skills Programme 2010). Kilimanjaro Tourism and What It Means for Local Porters and the Local Environment. *Journal of Ritsumeikan Social Sciences and Humanities, 4*, 1-12.

Peck, R. B., Lim, J. M., van Rooyen, H., Mukoma, W., Chepuka, L., Bansil, P. . . . Taegtmeyer, M. (2014). What should the ideal HIV self-test look like? A usability study of test prototypes in unsupervised HIV self-testing in Kenya, Malawi and South Africa. *AIDS Behaviour, 18 Suppl 4*, S422-432. Doi: 10.1007/s10461-014-0818-8

Prazuck, T., Karon, S., Gubavu, C. andre, J., Legall, J. M., Bouvet, E. . . . Pialoux, G. (2016). A finger-stick whole-blood HIV self- test as an HIV screening tool adapted to the public. *PloS ONE., 11*(2), e0146755. Retrieved from https:// Doi.org/10.1371/journal.pone.0146755https://www.ncbi.nlm.nih.gov/pmc/articles/PMC4755564/pdf/pone.0146755.pdf

Sarkar, A., Mburu, G., Shivkumar, P. V., Sharma, P., Campbell, F., Behera, J. . . . Mehra, S. (2016). Feasibility of supervised self-testing using an oral fluid-based HIV rapid testing method: a cross-sectional, mixed-method study among pregnant women in rural India. *Journal of International AIDS Society, 19*(1), 20993. Doi:10.7448/IAS.19.1.20993

Scott-Sheldon, L. A. J., Huedo-Medina, T. B., Warren, M. R., Johnson, B. T., & Carey, M. P. (2011). Efficacy of Behavioral Interventions to Increase Condom Use and Reduce Sexually Transmitted Infections: A Meta-Analysis, 1991 to 2010. *Journal of Acquired Immune Deficiency Syndromes, 58*(5).

Spielberg, F., Levine, R. O., & Weaver, M. (2004). Self-testing for HIV: a new option for HIV prevention? *Lancet Infectious Diseases, 4*, 640-646. Retrieved from http://ac.els-cdn.com/S1473309904011508/1-s2.0-S1473309904011508-main.pdf?_tid=a5fb659c-b430-11e4-b3e7-00000aab0f27&acdnat=1423908356_d7a4a45a0e07cb2432bb85acfbf3ba40

Staveteig, S., Wang, S., Hwad, S. K., Bradley, S. E. K., & Nybro, E. (2013). *Demographic Patterns of HIV Testing Uptake in sub-Saharan Africa*.

Suthar, A. B., Ford, N., Buchanan, P. J., Wong, V. J., Rajan, J. S., Saltzman, A. K., . . . Baggaley, R. C. (2013). Towards Universal Voluntary HIV Testing and Counselling A Systematic Review and Meta-Analysis of Community-Based Approaches. *PLoS Medicine, 10(8) :*(e1001496.). Doi:10.1371/journal.pmed.1001496

TACAIDS. (2018). *BOTTLENECKS AND CATCH-UP PLAN FOR ENGAGEMENT OF ADULT MEN AND ADOLESCENT BOYS IN HIV COUNSELLING AND TESTING IN TANZANIA*.

TENGIA-KESSY, A., & LYAMUYA, D. E. (2018). The utilization of voluntary counselling and testing services among bar waitresses in Kinondoni District, Dar es Salaam, Tanzania. *Tanzania Journal of Health Research, Volume 20,* (Number 3,), 1-8. Doi:10.4314/thrb.v20i3.1

The IeDEA and ART cohort collaborations. (2014). Immunodeficiency at the start of combination antiretroviral therapy in low-, middle- and high-income countries. *Journal of Acquired Immune Deficiency Syndromes, 65(1): e8–e16*. Doi:10.1097/QAI.0b013e3182a39979

Thirumurthy, H., Masters, S. H., Mavedzenge, S. N., Maman, S., Omanga, E., & Agot, K. (2016). Promoting male partner HIV testing and safer sexual decision making through secondary distribution of self-tests by HIV-negative female sex workers and women receiving antenatal and post-partum care in Kenya: a cohort study. *Lancet HIV, 3*, e266–274.

THIS. (2017). *TANZANIA HIV IMPACT SURVEY (THIS) 2016-2017: PRELIMINARY FINDINGS*.

Tonen-Wolyec, S., Batina-Agasa, S., Muwonga, J., Fwamba N'kulu, F., Mboumba Bouassa, R. S., & Belec, L. (2018). Evaluation of the practicability and virological performance of finger-stick whole blood HIV self-testing in French-speaking sub-Saharan Africa. *PLoS ONE, 13*(1), e0189475. Doi:10.1371/journal.pone.0189475.

UNAIDS. (2014). *A short Technical Update on Self-Testing for HIV.*

UNAIDS. (2017). UNAIDS Data

UNAIDS. (2018). *Global AIDS Update 2018: Miles To Go Closing Gaps Breaking Barriers Righting Injustices*. Retrieved from http://www.unaids.org/sites/default/files/media_asset/miles-to-go_en.pdf.

UNAIDS/WHO. (Critical Appraisal Skills Programme 2010). *Towards universal access scaling up priority HIV/AIDS interventions in the health sector-progress report*. Retrieved from Geneva:

The United Republic of Tanzania, & Ministry of Health and Social Welfare National AIDS Control Programme (NACP). (2012). *National Guidelines for Management of HIV and AIDS*. Dar es Salaam, Tanzania.

The United Republic of Tanzania, N. B. S. (2012). *2012 Tanzania Population and Housing Census* Retrieved from Dar es Salaam: http://www.nbs.go.tz/sensa/index.html

US Food and Drug Administration(US Food and Drug Administration(FDA)). (2012). *OraQuick In-Home HIV test summary of safety and effectiveness*. Retrieved from Silver Spring: FDA 2012.

van Rooyen, H., Tulloch, O., Mukoma, W., Makusha, T., Chepuka, L., Knight, L. C., . . . Taegtmeyer, M. (2015). What are the constraints and opportunities for HIVST scale-up in Africa? Evidence from Kenya, Malawi and South Africa. *Journal of the International Aids Society, 18*(1), 19445. Doi:10.7448/ias.18.1.19445

Wanyenze, R. K., Kamya, M. R., Fatch, R., Mayanja-Kizza, H., Baveewo, S., Sawires, S. . . . Hahn, J. A. (2011). Missed Opportunities for HIV Testing and Late-Stage Diagnosis among HIV-Infected Patients in Uganda. *PLoS ONE, 6*(7). Doi:10.1371/journal.pone.0021794

WHO. (2013). *Report on the first international symposium on self-testing for HIV: the legal, ethical, gender, human rights and public health implication of HIV self-testing scale-up*. Retrieved from http://apps.who.int/iris/bitstream/10665/85267/1/9789241505628_eng.pdf.

World Health Organization. (2015). *Consolidated guidelines on HIV testing services*. Retrieved from Geneva: World Health Organization. July 2015. : http://www.who.int/hiv/pub/guidelines/hiv-testing-services/en/

World Health Organization. (2016a). *Guidelines on HIV self-testing and partner notification: supplement to consolidated guidelines on HIV testing services*. Retrieved from France.

World Health Organization. (2016b). *Technical specification series for submission to WHO prequalification– Diagnostic Assessment. TSS-1: Human Immunodeficiency Virus (HIV) rapid diagnostic tests for professional and/or self-testing. 2016*. . . . Retrieved from http://apps.who.int/iris/bitstream/10665/251857/1/9789241511742- eng.pdf?ua=1

World Health Organization. (2016c). WHO recommends HIV self-testing Policy brief. December 2016. [Press release]. Retrieved from https://apps.who.int/iris/bitstream/10665/251549/1/WHO-HIV-2016.21-eng.pdf?ua=1

WHO & UNITAID. (2016). *Technology Landscape, HIV rapid diagnostic tests for self-testing*. Retrieved from http://www.who.int/hiv/pub/vct/hiv-self-testing-2016- second edition/en/

Zanolini, A., Chipungu, J., Vinikoor, M. J., Bosomprah, S., Mafwenko, M., Holmes, C. B., & Thirumurthy, H. (2017). HIV Self-Testing in Lusaka Province, Zambia: Acceptability, Comprehension of Testing Instructions and Individual Preferences for Self-Test Kit Distribution in a Population-Based Sample of Adolescents and Adults. *AIDS Research and Human Retroviruses*. Doi:10.1089/AID.2017.0156

CHAPTER EIGHT

8.0 General discussion, conclusions and recommendations

8.1. Introduction

The overall aim of this book was to systematically develop and evaluate a theory-based behaviour change intervention (BCI) to increase HIVST uptake and linkage to HIV prevention, care and treatment among FBWs and MCPs in Northern Tanzania. This chapter presents the general discussion, conclusions and recommendations based on the findings of the two sub-studies included in this book. Sub-study 1 (SS1) addressed book objective one, which was to systematically review the evidence on the effects of HIVST on the uptake of HIV testing, the yield of new HIV-positive diagnosis, social harms and linkage to ART treatment and barriers to and facilitators for HIVST uptake among adults in Africa. The results of SS1 informed the development of the theory-based BCI to increase HIVST uptake and linkage to HIV prevention, care and treatment described in Sub-study 2 (SS2).

Sub-study 2 (SS2) addressed book objectives two to four, which were: to explore perceptions of key informants, community members and target population and contextual and organizational factors related to HIVST to inform the development of the BCI. Besides, SS2 included the development of the BCI and evaluation of the acceptability, feasibility and fidelity of the BCI and its impact on FBWs and MCPs beliefs, attitudes and personal agency to increase HIVST uptake and linkage to HIV prevention, care and treatment.

8.2 Methodological aspects

Although methodological aspects of this book were presented in respective chapters, elaboration on issues related to study design, selection bias, information bias, reliability and qualitative study rigour, as potential sources of

Furthermore, a discussion on measures taken to minimize sources of bias are also presented.

8.2.1 Research design

The uncontrolled before-after study design was selected to be feasible to undertake with relatively low cost, simplicity and within a reasonable period compared to a RCT.

The main disadvantage of the before-after design is the lack of a comparison or control group. Therefore, it cannot establish the cause-effect relationship between exposure and the outcome; hence, the assumption of causal inference becomes less robust compared to a RCT. A limitation of before-after study designs relates the inability to consider temporal changes independent of the intervention. Other potential limitations include the individuals selected for study (most are not representative of the general population) and regression to the mean (a common statistical phenomenon in which extreme values on any measure at a point in time will be less extreme the next time it is measured) may occur (Ho et al., 2018).
Measures used to minimize these potential limitations were to make sure that the study tested the same persons before and after the intervention. However, the author acknowledges the potential of risk of unidentifiable confounders in the evaluation study findings **(Chapter Seven)**.

8.2.2 External validity and selection bias

External validity refers to the extent to which the study findings can be generalized to a large population (Ho et al., 2018). Selection bias may occur during enrolment or due to the refusal to participate or loss to follow-up leading to the difference in characteristics related to exposure or outcome under investigation between individuals who are selected to participate and those who are not selected to participate in the study. The evaluation study was conducted in an urban setting whereby participants were invited and consented to participate **(Chapter Seven).** One of the inclusion criteria was a participant who had not been tested for HIV in the past 3 months or more, or those who do not know their HIV status. We also considered the age

Based on the above-mentioned inclusion criteria, there is a possibility of selection bias because of inadequate representation of participants who have tested for HIV in less than 3 months, or those below 18 years of age who may be at high risk of HIV infection. Hence, the study findings will not be representative of those other groups who were not included and may not be generalizability to the general population.

The proportion of participants who refused to participate in the evaluation study **(Chapter Seven)** was low. Of 183 eligible participants who were contacted to participate in the BCI, four (n=4; 2.2%) refused to participate. To minimize any errors of selection bias, reasons for refusal to participate were collected at baseline.

8.2.3 Information bias

Information bias refers to systematic differences in the way information is obtained from study participants. Interview bias is one form of information bias that may influence the validity of the study findings.

Interviewer bias

Interviewer's bias refers to a systematic difference in the way information is collected from study participants. When the interviewer has prior knowledge about individual exposure or outcome status, interviewer bias might occur. To minimize the problem of interview bias, this book used a standardized questionnaire **(Chapter Seven)** and well-trained research assistants conducted interviews based on a standardized protocol for data collection. In addition, the data collection instruments were administered in Swahili, a language familiar to and well understood by all study participants. Further, the data collection instrument was pilot tested before the main study to ascertain the content and competency of research assistants. Based on the above measures, the possibility that the study findings could be explained by the effect on interviewer bias is unlikely.

Loss-to-follow up

Loss-to-follow up occurs when individuals who were initially enrolled in the study and after collection of the baseline information withdraw, or do not appear at follow-up visits. In the evaluation study, at 3-months follow-up, loss to follow-up was low.

To minimize the problem of loss-to-follow up, participants were asked to provide their phone number or the address of their place of work at baseline, and at follow-up, trained peers were asked to make calls or physical visits to schedule for follow-up visits. This procedure was very successful in reaching all participants during the follow-up period.

8.2.4 Reliability

A scale or test is reliable if measurements made under constant conditions are likely to provide the same results, with the assumption that no changes occur in the basic characteristics measured.

In this book, reliability was assessed using a Cronbach's alpha coefficient, which is a measure of internal consistency (Cronbach 1951). In this book, Cronbach's alpha coefficient had a reliability index ranging from 0.70 to 0.87, suggesting acceptable levels of internal consistency **(Chapter Seven)**.

8.2.5 Qualitative study rigour

In qualitative research, internal validity is crucial in ascertaining that the study findings are a true reflection of the experiences of study participants. Credibility is one strategy to achieve internal validity in qualitative research. In this book, the qualitative formative study **(Chapter Five)** ascertained credibility through triangulation and audit trail. Triangulation refers to the application of multiple procedures, sources of data, or persons in acquiring data (Spencer et al., 2003). Triangulation was achieved during data analysis using the Framework Method described in **Chapter Five**. Additionally, an audit trail, which refers to keeping meticulous records of the process of the study through the author's reflexive thoughts and notes taken during the study period, determined the high level of objectivity. In **Chapter Five** of this book, detailed descriptions of the context, recruitment of study participants, the data collection procedures and steps for data analysis are presented.

Further, the author is a native of the study setting, where the interviews took place and have a lived experience of the contextual setting and the culture of the interviewees.

Moreover, the author set aside time after every interview to hold discussions with the research assistants in order to come into agreement and understanding of the collected data. Finally, the principal investigator used the memos and interview summaries written immediately after the interviews as a 'recall tool' to reflect the times when the interviews took place.

8.3 General findings

Based on the findings from the SS1, there is moderate evidence that HIVST compared to standard HTS may increase the uptake of HIV among adults in SSA (Gichangi et al., 2016, Masters et al., 2016, Chanda et al., 2017, Ortblad et al., 2018). Furthermore, HIVST has the potential to increase the uptake of couples' HIV testing. In addition, offering HIVST with an optional home initiation of HIV care compared with HIVST with facility-based HIV care significantly increases the proportion of adults into initiating ART (MacPherson et al., 2014).

However, there is a concern about the impact of home initiation on longer-term retention in care, particularly among men (Conserve et al., 2018a). Finally, the reported incidences of intimate partner violence related to HIVST were rare, but caution should be observed among vulnerable and key populations (Masters et al., 2016, WHO 2016, Chanda et al., 2017, Ortblad et al., 2018).

Findings from the synthesis of evidence showed concerns of HIV stakeholders, the main ones being human right issues, lack of linkage to care, face-to-face counselling, lack of regulatory and quality assurance systems and quality of HIVST kits, which needs attention. Several studies have extensively reported on the stigma related to HIV and AIDS, reaching a common conclusion that HIV stigma is a major barrier to uptake of HIV testing. It is clear that HIV stigma still needs attention and must be reduced (MacPherson et al., 2011, Musheke et al., 2013, Kumwenda et al., 2014, Jennings et al., 2017, Johnson et al., 2017, Kumwenda et al., 2018). In this study, participants perceived that HIVST might reduce stigma related to HIV testing at a health facility.

Hence, future BCI to increase HIVST uptake should address the role of stigma to improve the HIVST uptake and linkage to HIV prevention, care and treatment.

So far, to author's knowledge, no studies have been conducted to evaluate the acceptability and feasibility of a theory-based BCI and its impact to increase HIVST uptake and linkage to HIV prevention, care and treatment among hard-to-reach populations in Northern Tanzania. The study findings have provided additional information about the development and evaluation of a theory-based BCI in an urban setting.

Since HIV-related behaviour is influenced by multiple determinants, no single theory is adequate to achieve behaviour change. Hence, it is important to combine different theoretical models when designing a BCI to promote HIVST uptake and linkage to HIV prevention, care and treatment.

The before-after study findings suggest the BCI was acceptable among FBWs and MCPs and feasible in the study setting. In addition, the trained peer-educators implemented the BCI with moderate to high levels of fidelity. Further, HIVST had the potential to reach those who have never tested for HIV before, particularly men.

Despite of the current findings, there is a need for pragmatic designs in experimental approaches such as a-RCT in the future to evaluate the efficacy of the BCI to increase HIVST uptake and linkage to HIV prevention, care and treatment.

8.4 Implications of the book findings

8.4.1 Public health implications of the findings

The application of the IBM and the PRECEDE-PROCEED model assisted in reaching a deeper understanding of the complexities of the inter-relationships of contextual factors to design and develop a theory-based BCI for hard to reach the population in Northern Tanzania.

The findings highlighted the importance of HIVST as an alternative and complementary HTS (WHO 2016, UNAIDS 2019). The knowledge generated from the systematic review and evidence synthesis on HIVST underscored the potential of HIVST to act as an option for HTS and that the uptake of HIVST is promising among adults in the general populations, sero discordant couples, high-risk populations, health care providers, HIV experts and HIV policy stakeholders in Africa, particularly in SSA. Importantly, HIVST has the potential to reach male partners through couples' HIV testing and those who have never tested for HIV before (WHO 2016, UNAIDS 2019).

Currently, in Tanzania, HIVST is not fully adopted as a complementary HIV testing option except for research purposes (Conserve et al., 2018a, TACAIDS 2018). Nonetheless, the high HIVST uptake observed in this study calls for HIV experts and policymakers in the country to see an opportunity to consider HIVST as HIV testing option. Additionally, these findings will inform future policy and program guidance and scale-up of HIVST in the country.

Despite the high HIVST uptake reported in this book, it is clear there are gaps for linking clients with preliminary positive HIVST results to health facilities for confirmatory testing and HIV care, treatment and support as per WHO recommendation (WHO 2016). For scalability of HIVST and linkage to care, treatment and support, planners should guard against supervised HIVST. The fundamental principle for HIVST is to allow the choice of users to test without the presence of a counsellor, or a health worker (Asiimwe et al., 2014, Wong et al., 2014, Perez et al., 2016, Smith et al., 2016, Indravudh et al., 2018).

A key area of contention related to HIVST is lack of counselling – an inherent of HIVST and poor linkage of care post-testing (Mavedzenge et al., 2013, Makusha et al., 2015, van Rooyen et al., 2015, Mavedzenge et al., 2016, Gagnon et al., 2018). Individuals and HIV experts in the formative qualitative study agreed that the gap might lead to missing or delay treatment among HIV positive individuals. To address these concerns this book suggests areas for future research (see 8.6 below).

8.5 General Conclusion

HIV and AIDS is still a public health problem globally and more significantly in SSA, including in Tanzania. Results from the systematic review suggest moderate-quality evidence that HIVST has the potential to provide an innovative strategy to increase uptake of HIV testing and increase awareness of HIV status among undiagnosed adults in Africa, particularly in SSA. If adopted as a complimentary HTS option, HIVST could facilitate early detection, early care, treatment and prevention and maybe pivotal in providing an invaluable tool for health authorities of African governments to increase access to HIV care, treatment and prevention to achieve the "95-95-95" global target by the year 2030 (UNAIDS 2017, UNAIDS 2019). Additionally, a theory-based BCI was acceptable among the target population, with high levels of fidelity leading to HIVST uptake and linkage to HIV prevention care and treatment.

Results from this book show that there are potential opportunities to implement a theory-based BCI if proper strategies and/or methods are incorporated in the design and development of the intervention that addresses all negative beliefs, including potential barriers and facilitators that may hinder or promote HIVST uptake.

Further, different strategies and approaches that would facilitate a successful HIVST uptake, including the use of mobile applications, such as phone calls and short messages services (SMS) to facilitate the preferred support, community-based information campaign using trained opinion leaders, peer networks and effective communication channels, should be employed. Importantly, the study findings indicated that a BCI that addresses potential barriers to HIVST has the potential to increase HIVST uptake, reduce perceived stigma and increase linkage to HTS.
The development of a BCI to increase HIVST uptake and linkage to HIV prevention, care and treatment should aim to enhance locally appropriate facilitators unique to specific local contexts, to ensure high acceptability, uptake and feasibility of a theory-based BCI to increase HIVST uptake and linkage to HIV prevention, care and treatment among MCPs and FBWs in Northern Tanzania.

8.6. General Recommendations

To optimize the scaling-up of HIVST as an alternative and complementary HTS among hard to reach the population in Tanzania, it is important to design BCIs that would mitigate the barriers for HIVST uptake and linkage to HIV prevention, care and treatment. Thus, this book proposes the following recommendations

(a) A randomized clinical trial intervention is warranted to evaluate the efficacy of a theory-based BCI to increase of HIVST uptake and linkage to testing among targeted populations. However, given the challenges of conducting clinical trials, an alternative discrete choice experiment (DCE) may be useful for generating information for informing HTS policy decisions about HIVST.

(b) Innovative follow-up strategies to HIV prevention, care, treatment and support are needed in this setting to encourage linkage to care post-testing.

8.7 Areas for future research

In addition to the application of the findings presented in this book, several key areas that may direct future research on HIVST are presented as follows:

(a) To determine the effectiveness of behavioural interventions to reduce HIV-related risk-behaviours among key populations (i.e., men having sex with men (MSM), people who inject drugs (PWIDs), or people who use drugs (PWUDs), female sex workers (FSWs), young adolescent girls and women and vulnerable groups in high HIV prevalence settings.

(b) To determine the efficacy of a theory-based BCI in detecting previously undiagnosed HIV infection, or the number of repeat non-testers and linkage to care following a reactive HIVST test result or a confirmatory positive test in high HIV prevalence settings.

(c) To determine the retention in care among participants identified HIV-positive and linkage to prevention services among those with negative results (e.g. male circumcision) and social harms from HIVST.

References

Asiimwe, S., J. Oloya, X. Song and C. C. Whalen (2014). "Accuracy of un-supervised versus provider-supervised self-administered HIV testing in Uganda: A randomized implementation trial." AIDS Behavior **18**(12): 2477-2484.

Chanda, M. M., K. F. Ortblad, M. Mwale, S. Chongo, C. Kanchele, N. Kamungoma, et al. (2017). "HIV self-testing among female sex workers in Zambia: A cluster randomized controlled trial." PLoS Medicine **14**(11): e1002442.

Choko, A. T., E. L. Corbett, N. Stallard, H. Maheswaran, A. Lepine, C. C. Johnson, et al. (2019). "HIV self-testing alone or with additional interventions, including financial incentives, and linkage to care or prevention among male partners of antenatal care clinic attendees in Malawi: An adaptive multi-arm, multi-stage cluster randomized trial." PLoS Medicine **16**(1): e1002719.

Choko, A. T., N. Desmond, E. L. Webb, K. Chavula, S. Napierala-Mavedzenge, C. A. Gaydos, et al. (2011). "The Uptake and Accuracy of Oral Kits for HIV Self-Testing in High HIV Prevalence Setting: A Cross-Sectional Feasibility Study in Blantyre, Malawi." PLoS Medicine **8**(10).

Choko, A. T., M. K. Kumwenda, C. C. Johnson, D. W. Sakala, M. C. Chikalipo, K. Fielding, et al. (2017). "Acceptability of woman-delivered HIV self-testing to the male partner, and additional interventions: a qualitative study of antenatal care participants in Malawi." Journal of the International Aids Society **20**(1): 1-10.

Choko, A. T., P. MacPherson, E. L. Webb, B. A. Willey, H. Feasy, R. Sambakunsi, et al. (2015). "Uptake, Accuracy, Safety, and Linkage into Care over Two Years of Promoting Annual Self-Testing for HIV in Blantyre, Malawi: A Community-Based Prospective Study." PLoS Medicine **12**(9): e1001873.

Conserve, D. F., D. Alemu, T. Yamanis, S. Maman and L. Kajula (2018). "He Told Me to Check My Health": A Qualitative Exploration of Social Network Influence on Men's HIV Testing Behavior and HIV Self-Testing Willingness in Tanzania." American Journal of Men's Health.

Conserve, D. F., K. E. Muessig, L. L. Maboko, S. Shirima, M. N. Kilonzo, S. Maman, et al. (2018). "Mate Yako Afya Yako: Formative research to develop the Tanzania HIV self-testing education and promotion (Tanzania STEP) project for men." PLoS ONE.

Cronbach, L. J. (1951). "Coefficient alpha and the internal structure of tests." Psychometrika **16**: 297-334.

Gagnon, M., M. French, and Y. Hebert (2018). "The HIV self-testing debate: where do we stand?" BMC Int Health Hum Rights **18**(1): 5.

Gichangi, A., J. Wambua, A. Gohole, S. Mutwiwa, R. Njogu, E. Bazant, et al. (2016). Provision of oral HIV self-test Kits triples uptake of HIV testing among male partners of antenatal care clients:

results of a randomized trial in Kenya. 21st International AIDS Conference;18-22 July, Durban, South Africa.

Ho, A. M. H., R. Phelan, G. B. Mizubuti, J. A. C. Murdoch, S. Wickett, A. K. Ho, et al. (2018). "Bias in Before-After Studies: Narrative Overview for Anesthesiologists." Anesthesia Analgesia **126**(5): 1755-1762.

Indravudh, P. P., A. T. Choko and E. L. Corbett (2018). "Scaling up HIV self-testing in sub-Saharan Africa: a review of technology, policy, and evidence." Current Opinion Infectious Diseases **31**(1): 14-24.

Indravudh, P. P., E. L. Sibanda, M. d'Elbee, M. K. Kumwenda, B. Ringwald, G. Maringwa, et al. (2017). "'I will choose when to test, where I want to test': investigating young people's preferences for HIV self-testing in Malawi and Zimbabwe." AIDS **31 Suppl 3**: S203-S212.

Jennings, L., D. F. Conserve, J. Merrill, L. Kajula, J. Iwelunmor, S. Linnemayr, et al. (2017). "Perceived Cost Advantages and Disadvantages of Purchasing HIV Self- Testing Kits among Urban Tanzanian Men: An Inductive Content Analysis." Journal of AIDS & Clinical Research **08**(08).

Johnson, C. C., C. Kennedy, V. A. Fonner, N. Siegfried, C. Figueroa, S. Dalal, et al. (2017). "Examining the effects of HIV self-testing compared to standard HIV testing services: a systematic review and meta-analysis." Journal of the International Aids Society **20**(1).

Kumwenda, M., A. Munthali, M. Phiri, D. Mwale, T. Gutteberg, E. MacPherson, et al. (2014). "Factors shaping initial decision-making to self-test amongst cohabiting couples in urban Blantyre, Malawi." AIDS Behavior **18 Suppl 4**: S396-404.

Kumwenda, M. K., E. L. Corbett, J. Chikovore, M. Phiri, D. Mwale, A. T. Choko, et al. (2018). "Discordance, Disclosure and Normative Gender Roles: Barriers to Couple Testing Within a Community-Level HIV Self-Testing Intervention in Urban Blantyre, Malawi." AIDS Behav **22**(8): 2491-2499.

MacPherson, P., D. G. Lalloo, E. L. Webb, H. Maheswaran, A. T. Choko, S. D. Makombe, et al. (2014). "Effect of Optional Home Initiation of HIV Care Following HIV Self-testing on Antiretroviral Therapy Initiation Among Adults in Malawi: A Randomized Clinical Trial." Jama **312**(4): 372-379.

MacPherson, P., E. L. Webb, A. T. Choko, N. Desmond, K. Chavula, S. Napierala Mavedzenge, et al. (2011). "Stigmatising Attitudes among People Offered Home-Based HIV Testing and Counselling in Blantyre, Malawi: Construction and Analysis of a Stigma Scale." PLoS ONE **6**(10): e26814.

Makusha, T., L. Knight, M. Taegtmeyer, O. Tulloch, A. Davids, J. Lim, et al. (2015). "HIV Self-Testing Could "Revolutionize Testing in South Africa, but It Has Got to Be Done Properly": Perceptions of Key Stakeholders." PLoS ONE **10**(3): e0122783.

Masters, S. H., K. Agot, B. Obonyo, S. Napierala Mavedzenge, S. Maman and H. Thirumurthy (2016). "Promoting Partner Testing and Couples Testing through Secondary Distribution of HIV Self-Tests: A Randomized Clinical Trial." PLoS Medicine **13**(11): e1002166.

Mavedzenge, S. N., R. Baggaley and E. L. Corbett (2013). "A review of self-testing for HIV: research and policy priorities in a new era of HIV prevention." Clinical Infectious Diseases **57**(1): 126-138.

Mavedzenge, S. N., E. Sibanda, Y. Mavengere, J. Dirawo, K. Hatzold, O. Mugurungi, et al. (2016). Acceptability, feasibility, and preference for HIV self-testing in Zimbabwe. 21st International AIDS Conference, Durban, South Africa, July 18-22, 2016.

Musheke, M., H. Ntalasha, S. Gari, O. McKenzie, V. Bond, A. Martin-Hilber, et al. (2013). "A systematic review of qualitative findings on factors enabling and deterring uptake of HIV testing in Sub-Saharan Africa." BMC Public Health **13**: 220.

Ortblad, K. F., M. M. Chanda, D. K. Musoke, T. Ngabirano, M. Mwale, A. Nakitende, et al. (2018). "Acceptability of HIV self-testing to support pre-exposure prophylaxis among female sex workers in Uganda and Zambia: results from two randomized controlled trials." BMC Infectious Diseases **18**(1): 503.

Perez, G. M., S. J. Steele, I. Govender, G. Arellano, A. Mkwamba, M. Hadebe, et al. (2016). "Supervised oral HIV self-testing is accurate in rural KwaZulu-Natal, South Africa." Tropical Medicine and International Health **21**(6): 759–767.

Smith, P., M. Wallace and L. G. Bekker (2016). "Adolescents' experience of a rapid HIV self- && testing device in youth-friendly clinic settings in Cape Town South Africa: a cross-sectional community-based usability study. ." Journal of International AIDS Society **19:1 – 6.**(1): 21111.

Spencer, L., J. Ritchie and W. O'Connor (2003). Carrying out qualitative analysis. *Qualitative research practice: a guide for social science students and researchers*. J. Ritchie and J. Lewis. London/Thousand Oaks, CA/New Delhi, Sage Publications, pp. 219-62.

TACAIDS (2018). BOTTLENECKS AND CATCH-UP PLAN FOR ENGAGEMENT OF ADULT MEN AND ADOLESCENT BOYS IN HIV COUNSELING AND TESTING IN TANZANIA., TANZANIA COMMISSION FOR AIDS(TACAIDS)2018.

UNAIDS (2017). "UNAIDS Data ".

van Rooyen, H., O. Tulloch, W. Mukoma, T. Makusha, L. Chepuka, L. C. Knight, et al. (2015). "What are the constraints and opportunities for HIVST scale-up in Africa? Evidence from Kenya, Malawi and South Africa." Journal of the International Aids Society **18**(1): 19445.

Wong, V., C. Johnson, E. Cowan, M. Rosenthal, R. Peeling, M. Miralles, et al. (2014). "HIV Self-Testing in Resource-Limited Settings: Regulatory and Policy Considerations." AIDS Behavior **18 Suppl 4**: S415-421.

World Health Organization (2016). Guidelines on HIV self-testing and partner notification: supplement to consolidated guidelines on HIV testing services. France., World Health Organization, Geneva 27, Switzerland.: 1-104.

APPENDICES:

Appendix A: Describing details of search strategy		
Concept		Search terms
Population	Adults	"adult"[MeSH Terms] OR (adult[All Fields] OR adulterant[All Fields] OR adulterate[All Fields] OR adulterated[All Fields] OR adulteration[All Fields] OR adulterations[All Fields] OR adultery[All Fields] OR adulthood[All Fields] OR adulticidal[All Fields] OR adultorum[All Fields] OR adults[All Fields])) OR ("young adult"[MeSH Terms] OR young adults[Text Word])) OR (young adult[All Fields] OR young adulthood[All Fields] OR young adults[All Fields])) OR ("middle aged"[MeSH Terms] OR middle aged[Text Word])) OR ("aged"[MeSH Terms] OR aged[Text Word])) OR ("aged, 80 and over"[MeSH Terms] OR aged, 80 and over[Text Word])
Intervention	HIV self-testing	"HIV Infections" OR "HIV"[MeSH] OR "hiv"[tiab] OR hiv-1*[tiab] OR hiv-2*[tiab] OR hiv1[tiab] OR hiv2[tiab] OR hiv infect*[tiab] OR human immunodeficiency virus[tiab] OR human immunedeficiency virus[tiab] OR human immuno-deficiency virus[tiab] OR human immune-deficiency virus[tiab] OR (human immun*[tiab] AND deficiency virus[tiab]) OR acquired immunodeficiency syndrome[tiab] OR acquired immunedeficiency syndrome[tiab] OR acquired immuno-deficiency syndrome[tiab] OR acquired immune-deficiency syndrome[tiab] OR (acquired immun*[tiab] AND deficiency syndrome[tiab]) OR "sexually transmitted diseases, Viral"[MeSH:noexp]) AND self-testing; self-test* HIV self-testing; HIVST; "diagnostic self-evaluation" [MeSH]; "self care" [MeSH]; "self-administration"[MeSH]; "self-administration"[MeSH] "testing";"counseling" NOT (animals [mh] NOT humans [mh]).
Comparison	HIV testing standard of care	(testing AND (standard of care)) OR (provider-administered test) OR (provider-initiated test) OR (provider-initiated testing) OR (client-initiated testing) OR (client-initiated test) OR (community-based HIV testing) OR (home-based HIV testing) OR (house-based HIV testing) OR (door-to-door-based HIV testing) OR (mobile HIV testing) OR (HIV testing campaign) OR (bar-based HIV testing) OR (workplace HIV testing) OR (business-based HIV testing) OR (church-based HIV testing) OR (outreach-based HIV testing)
Outcome	Uptake of HIV testing Yield Linkage	Uptake OR (uptake of care) OR Yield OR (HIV prevalence) OR (HIV Seroprevalence)[mh] OR (HIV seroprevalence) OR (HIV positivity) OR (social Harm) OR (HIV linkage) OR (linkage to care)
	ART	(antiretroviral therapy, highly active[MeSH] OR anti-retroviral agents[MeSH] OR antiviral agents[MeSH:NoExp] OR ((anti[tiab]) AND (hiv[tiab])) OR antiretroviral*[tiab] OR ((anti[tiab]) AND (retroviral*[tiab])) OR HAART[tiab] OR ((anti[tiab]) AND (acquired immunodeficiency[tiab])) OR ((anti[tiab]) AND (acquired immuno-deficiency[tiab])) OR

		((anti[tiab]) AND (acquired immune-deficiency[tiab])) OR ((anti[tiab]) AND (acquired immun*[tiab]) AND (deficiency[tiab])))
	CD 4 count	"antigens"[MeSH Terms] OR antigens[Text Word]) OR (antigen[All Fields] OR antigen/cea[All Fields] OR antigen/factor[All Fields] OR antigen's[All Fields] OR antigenetic[All Fields] OR antigenic[All Fields] OR antigenically[All Fields] OR antigenicity[All Fields] OR antigenotoxic[All Fields] OR antigens[All Fields] OR antigens/immunology[All Fields] OR antigensynthesis[All Fields] OR antigentically[All Fields])) OR CD4[All Fields]) OR ("t-lymphocytes"[MeSH Terms] OR T-Cell[Text Word])) OR receptors[All Fields]) OR ("cd4 antigens"[MeSH Terms] OR CD4 receptors[Text Word])) OR ("t-lymphocytes"[MeSH Terms] OR T Cell[Text Word])) OR T[All Fields]
	Social harm	"Social harm"
udy design	RCT	AND (randomized controlled trial [pt] OR controlled clinical trial [pt] OR randomized [tiab] OR placebo [tiab] OR drug therapy [sh] OR randomly [tiab] OR trial [tiab] OR groups [tiab]) AND quasi-experimental[MeSH Terms]; after[All Fields] OR (pre[All Fields] AND post[All Fields] AND ("research design"[MeSH Terms] OR test[Text Word]))) OR controlled[All Fields]) OR ("interrupted time series analysis"[MeSH Terms] OR interrupted time series[Text Word])) OR CBA[All Fields] " research design"[MeSH Terms] OR test[Text word]
	Quasi-experimental	
	Pre and post	
	Controlled before/after	
	Interrupted time series	
frica		Africa [MeSH Terms] OR Africa [All Fields] (''Africa''[MeSH] OR Africa*[tw] OR Algeria[tw] OR Angola[tw] OR Benin[tw] OR Botswana[tw] OR ''Burkina Faso''[tw] OR Burundi[tw] OR Cameroon[tw] OR ''Canary Islands''[tw] OR ''Cape Verde''[tw] OR ''Central African Republic''[tw] OR Chad[tw] OR Comoros[tw] OR Congo[tw] OR ''Democratic Republic of Congo''[tw] OR Djibouti[tw] OR Egypt[tw] OR ''Equatorial Guinea''[tw] OR Eritrea[tw] OR Ethiopia[tw] OR Gabon[tw] OR Gambia[tw] OR Ghana[tw] OR Guinea[tw] OR ''GuineaBissau''[tw] OR ''Ivory Coast''[tw] OR ''Cote d'Ivoire''[tw] OR Jamahiriya[tw] OR Jamahiriya[tw] OR Kenya[tw] OR Lesotho[tw] OR Liberia[tw] OR Libya[tw] OR Libya[tw] OR Madagascar[tw] OR Malawi[tw] OR Mali[tw] OR Mauritania[tw] OR Mauritius[tw] OR Mayotte[tw] OR Morocco[tw] OR Mozambique[tw] OR Mozambique[tw] OR Namibia[tw] OR Niger[tw] OR Nigeria[tw] OR Principe[tw] OR Reunion[tw] OR Rwanda[tw] OR ''SaoTome''[tw] OR Senegal[tw] OR Seychelles[tw] OR ''SierraLeone''[tw] OR Somalia[tw] OR ''South Africa''[tw] OR ''St Helena''[tw] OR Sudan[tw] OR Swaziland[tw] OR Tanzania[tw] OR Togo[tw] OR

	Tunisia[tw] OR Uganda[tw] OR ''Western Sahara''[tw] OR Zaire[tw] OR Zambia[tw] OR Zimbabwe[tw] OR ''Central Africa''[tw] OR ''Central African''[tw] OR ''West Africa''[tw] OR ''West African''[tw] OR ''Western Africa''[tw] OR ''Western African''[tw] OR ''East Africa''[tw] OR ''East African''[tw] OR ''Eastern Africa''[tw] OR "Eastern African"[tw] OR "Northern Africa" [tw] OR ''Southern Africa''[tw] OR ''Southern African''[tw] OR ''sub Saharan Africa''[tw] OR ''sub Saharan African''[tw] OR ''sub-Saharan Africa''[tw] OR ''sub-Saharan African''[tw]) NOT (''guinea pig''[tw] OR ''guinea pigs''[tw] OR 'aspergillums Niger''[tw])

Appendix B: Sample of data extraction form (Systematic review)

DATA EXTRACTION FORM

STUDY ID:"################################" " " Date form completed:"________________"

Reviewer's initials [ ]

Part 1: COVER SHEET

Study Title: [ ]

Authors: [ ]

Journal: [ ]

Contact details: [ ]

Language:...

Citation: [ ]

"

"""""""""""""""""""Part 2: STUDY CHARACTERISTICS

Publication Year:............................Country of Study:.........................

Eligibility: (use attached check list) Confirm eligibility for review? Yes [ ] No [ ]

Decision taken: Included [ ] Excluded [ ] Pending [ ]

If not included, give reasons why: [ ]

DO NOT PROCEED IF STUDY EXCLUDED FROM REVIEW

Methods:

Aim(s) of the study: [ ]

Ethical approval obtained: Yes [ ] No [ ] Unclear [ ] Not reported [ ]

Study design:		Study population:		Total numbers:
Observational:		Adults	[ ]	[ ]
Cross-sectional	[ ]	Males	[ ]	[ ]
Cohort-study	[ ]	Females	[ ]	[ ]
Pre/post	[ ]	Both	[ ]	[ ]

1"

"

Appendix C: Search strategy (Qualitative evidence synthesis)	
S5	Facilitator* OR motivator*
S4	Barrier* OR challeng* OR obstacle* OR Imped* OR experience*
S3	Counsel*OR test*OR HIV test*OR self-test* OR HIV self-testing OR unsupervised self-testing OR supervised self-testing
S2	Africa* OR northern africa* OR western africa* OR eastern africa*OR southern africa* OR sub saharan africa* OR SSA
S1	Adult* OR young adult*OR adolescent* OR middle age* OR aged OR "aged, 80 and over"

Appendix D: Sample of data extraction form (Qualitative evidence synthesis)

Data collection method:						
Survey						
In-depth interviews						
Focus group discussions						
Group discussions						
Other(s)						
Outcome(s)						
Thematic analysis						
Overall perception of uptake of HIV self testing						
Checklist for qualitative studies						
	Description and assessment			Comments	Location in text/source	
Type of qualitative study	Participant observation					
	Open-ended interviews					
	Structured interviews					
	Others(specify):					
Theoretical approach	Appropriate		Inappropriate		Not sure	
1. Is a qualitative approach appropriate?						
For example						
(a) Does the research questin seek to understand process or structures ,or illuminate subjective experinces or meanings?						
(b) Could a quantitative approach better have addressed the research question?						
2. Is the study clear in what it seeks to do?						
	Clear		Unclear		Mixed	
For example						
(i)Is the purpose of the study discussed: aims/objectives/research(s)?						
(ii)Is there adequate/appropriate refrenece to the literature?						
(iii) Are underpinning values/assumptions/theory discussed?						
Study design						
3.How defensible/ rigorous is the research design/ methodology?						
	Defensible		Indefensible		Not sure	
For example						
(a) Is the design appropriate to the resarch question?						
(b) Is a rationale given for using a qualitative approach?						
(c) Are there clear accounts of the rationale/justification for the sampling,data collection and data analysis techniques used?						
(d) Is the selectin of cases/sampling startergy theoretically justified?						
Data collection	Appropriate		Inappropriate		Not sure/inadequately reported	
4.How well was the data collection carried out?						
For example						
(i) Are the data collection methods clearly described?						
(ii) Where the approprtaite data collected to address the research question(s)?						
(iii)Was the data collection and record keeping systematic?						
Trustworthiness	Clearly described		Unclear		Not described	
5. Is the role of the researcher clearly described?						
For example						
(a)Has the relationship between the researcher and participants been adequately considered?						

Appendix E: PRISMA Checklist			
Section/topic	**#**	**Checklist item**	**Reported on page #**
TITLE			
Title	1	Identify the report as a systematic review, meta-analysis, or both.	
ABSTRACT			
Structured summary	2	Provide a structured summary including, as applicable: background; objectives; data sources; study eligibility criteria, participants, and interventions; study appraisal and synthesis methods; results; limitations; conclusions and implications of key findings; systematic review registration number.	
INTRODUCTION			
Rationale	3	Describe the rationale for the review in the context of what is already known.	
Objectives	4	Provide an explicit statement of questions being addressed with reference to participants, interventions, comparisons, outcomes, and study design (PICOS).	
METHODS			
Protocol and registration	5	Indicate if a review protocol exists, if and where it can be accessed (e.g., Web address), and, if available, provide registration information including registration number.	
Eligibility criteria	6	Specify study characteristics (e.g., PICOS, length of follow-up) and report characteristics (e.g., years considered, language, publication status) used as criteria for eligibility, giving rationale.	
Information sources	7	Describe all information sources (e.g., databases with dates of coverage, contact with study authors to identify additional studies) in the search and date last searched.	
Search	8	Present full electronic search strategy for at least one database, including any limits used, such that it could be repeated.	
Study selection	9	State the process for selecting studies (i.e., screening, eligibility, included in systematic review, and, if applicable, included in the meta-analysis).	
Data collection process	10	Describe method of data extraction from reports (e.g., piloted forms, independently, in duplicate) and any processes for obtaining and confirming data from investigators.	
Data items	11	List and define all variables for which data were sought (e.g., PICOS, funding sources) and any assumptions and simplifications made.	
Risk of bias in individual studies	12	Describe methods used for assessing risk of bias of individual studies (including specification of whether this was done at the study or outcome level), and how this information is to be used in any data synthesis.	
Summary measures	13	State the principal summary measures (e.g., risk ratio, difference in means).	

thesis of results	14	Describe the methods of handling data and combining results of studies, if done, including measures of consistency (e.g., I^2) for each meta-analysis.	

Appendix F
IN-DEPTH INTERVIEW GUIDE FOR KEY INFORMANTS (HIV EXPERTS)

ENGLISH VERSION: The Project title: "A multi-component theory-based behaviour change intervention to increase HIV Self–testing uptake and linkage to HIV prevention, care, and treatment among hard to reach adults in Northern Tanzania".

INTRODUCTION [15 min]:

A. Introduce yourself to the interviewee

1.1 Introduce in-depth interview/focus group purpose and objectives

The main purpose of this research is to know if HIV self-testing (HIVST) can be offered to participants at high risk of HIV infection and whether this intervention would improve HIV testing. The Social Behavioural Science Training Program through Duke University in the United States sponsors this study. During the interview, I will ask you different questions about your thoughts on HIVST. Please keep in mind that *there are no right or wrong answers*, we are only interested in what you think. You may refuse to answer any questions or end your participation at any time.

1.2 INTERVIEWER: Distribute and review the informed consent form

Your rights as a participant in this research study are important. I would like to review the Informed Consent Form and ask you to sign it. There are 2 copies, one that I will keep and the other is yours.

Interviewer:

Read the consent form verbatim

Before each new heading ask if there are any questions.

Ask to sign one copy of the form

1.3 Collect signed consent forms and record respondent ID

Interviewer:

Collect the signed informed consent form from the interviewee.

Sign and date the consent form.

Put a unique ID on both the consent form and the in-depth interview guide

Date: _ _/_ _/_ _ _ _

A: PERSONAL INFORMATION [5 MIN]

Participant ID: [ ]

Enrolment date:

Interviewer:

Place of interview:

Age:

Gender:

Education level:

Occupation:

Currently working(yes/no):

Religion:

Residence:

B: HIVST ***as a delivery service in Tanzania***

I would like to explore your thoughts about **HIV SELF TESTING (HIVST),** which is not currently available in Tanzania but might be possible at some point in the future. When I talk about self-testing, I
want you to think about HIV test kits that may be available for purchase at a pharmacy, with tests performed by the client usually at a private place.

C: Knowledge of HIVST.

Q1: What is the first thing that comes to mind when you hear the phrase HIVST?

[**Probe:** Source of information; availability of adequate information; different communication channels to disseminate the knowledge, etc.].

Q2: If we offer HIVST, do you think you will be interested? Why or why not?

Q3: What are the benefits that might result from people doing HIVST?
[**Probe:** Privacy of testing; confidentiality of test results; reduced stigma; minimal physical contact with a counsellor, fewer needle pricks, ability to get at high-risk people, increase disclosure among couples, etc.].

D: Service delivery approaches:
Q4: With your experience in HIV Testing Services (HTS), what is your opinion on how best to deliver HIVST in the community? [**Probe:** door-to-door;pharmacy-based;workplace-based;internet-based; pre-exposure prophylaxis;vending-machine;kiosks;integrated services; partner-delivery; facility-based; community-based groups/peers;etc]

E: Linkage strategies post-self-testing
Q5: With your experience in HTS, what is your opinion on how best to follow-up clients and link them to HIV prevention, care and treatment post-self-testing [**Probe:** peers/outreach workers; home-based; use of brochures/flyers; telephone hotlines; mobile-phone text message services; internet/computer-based applications; vouchers/coupons incentives; appointment cards/referral-letters, etc.].

F: Monitoring of HIVST
Q6: With your experience in HTS, what is your opinion on how best to collect information on how effective an HIVST programme is?[**Probe:** calls to HIVST hotlines; community-based surveillance systems; facility-level testing registers; internet/mobile phone surveys; financial/in-kind incentives, etc.].

G: Barriers to, and facilitators for HIVST
Q7: What do you think will motivate or impede people who may decide to use self-testing?[**Probe:** lack of policy on self-testing; lack of regulatory systems for HIVST; lack of knowledge on HIVST; lack of counsellor assistance; lack of the HIVST kits; fear of HIV-positive results, inability to perform the testing, cost of buying HIVST kits, etc.].

Q8: What do you think will make it easy to implement HIVST in the community? [**Probe:** training on HIVST; availability of HIVST kits, demonstrations on how to do HIVST, simple /clear instruction, language, etc.].

Q9: Think back to the barriers that we have discussed. What do you think could be done to overcome any of the barriers?

Q10: In your opinion, how do you think HIVST should be conducted?
[**Probe:** how will this be possible? Someone gets an HIVST kit, and then go to test in privacy, then what next? Would they prefer self-testing at a clinic or alternative sites? Provision of assistance from counsellors? A need for post-test counselling? Confirmatory test for HIV positive results? Referral of HIV-positives to care & treatment? , the role of opinion leaders in promoting HIVST, channels of communication, etc.].

Q11: If HIVST was to be offered into the community, is there anything that makes it very difficult to promote HIVST or convince someone to use HIVST? Is there anything?

CONCLUSION:
Interviewer: Now I have asked you all my questions. Do you have additional comments about HIVST or advice on how best to conduct an HIVST intervention for at high-risk adults?

Appendix G

INTERVIEW GUIDE FOR FOCUS GROUP DISCUSSION (FGD)-ENGLISH VERSION: The Project title: "A multi-component theory-based behaviour change intervention to increase HIV Self–testing uptake and linkage to HIV prevention, care, and treatment among hard to reach adults in Northern Tanzania".

1 **INTRODUCTION [15 min]:**

. **A. Introduce yourself to the interviewee**

1.1 Introduce in-depth interview/focus group purpose and objectives

The main purpose of this research is to know if HIV self-testing (HIVST) can be offered to participants at high risk of HIV infection and whether this intervention would improve HIV testing. During the interview, I will ask you different questions about your thoughts on HIV testing in general and HIV self-testing in particular. Please keep in mind that *there are no right or wrong answers*, we are only interested in what you think. We will not offer HIV testing as part of this FGD, and you do not have to tell us about any HIV test results you may have received previously. You may refuse to answer any questions or end your participation at any time.

1.2 INTERVIEWER: Distribute and review the informed consent form

Your rights as a participant in this research study are important. We would like to review the Informed Consent Form and ask you to sign it. There are 2 copies, one that we will keep and the other is yours.

Interviewer:

Read the consent form verbatim

Before each new heading, ask if there are any questions.

Ask to sign one copy of the form

1.3 Collect signed consent forms and record respondent ID

Interviewer:

Collect the signed informed consent form from the interviewee.

Sign and date the consent form.

Put a unique ID on both the consent form and the in-depth interview guide

Date: _ _/_ _/_ _ _ _

A: PERSONAL INFORMATION [5 MIN]

Participant ID: [ ]

Enrolment date:

Interviewer:

Place of interview:

Age:

Gender:

Education level:

Occupation:

Currently working(yes/no):

Religion:

Residence:

HIV self-testing as a delivery service in Tanzania

Now we would like to explore your thoughts about **HIV SELF TESTING (HIVST),** which is not currently available in Tanzania but might be possible in the future. When I talk about self-testing, I want you to think about HIV test kits that may be available for purchase at a pharmacy, with tests performed by the client usually at a private place.

B: Knowledge of HIVST.
Q1: What is the first thing that comes to mind when you hear the phrase **HIVST**?
[**Probe:** Source of information; availability of adequate information; different communication channels to disseminate the knowledge, etc.].

Q2: If we offer **HIVST**, do you think you will be interested? Why or why not?

C: Experiential attitude towards HIVST
Q3: How do you feel about the idea of HIVST [**Probe:** what do they like/dislike about HIVST; what do they hate about **HIVST**, etc.].

D: Instrumental attitude towards HIVST
Q4: What are the positive consequences that might result from you doing HIVST [**Probe:** advantages of doing HIVST].

Q5: What are the benefits that might result from doing HIVST?
[**Probe:** Privacy of testing; confidentiality of test results; reduced stigma; minimal physical contact with a counsellor, fewer needle pricks, ability to get at high-risk people, increase disclosure among couples, etc.].

Q6: What are the negative consequences that might result from you doing HIVST [**Probe:** disadvantages of doing HIVST, fear of negative social consequences post HIV positive results; stigma & discrimination; involving other family members; etc.].

E: Normative influence on HIVST
Q7: What would people who are important to you think you should do regarding HIVST? [**Probe:** spouse/live-in partner willingness to self-test; significant others willingness to self-test (e.g., father, mother, relatives, religious leaders, peers, local leaders, etc.].

Q8: What would people we have just discussed think about HIVST? [**Probe:** spouse/live-in partner willingness to self-test; significant others willingness to self-test (e.g., father, mother, relatives, religious leaders, peers, local leaders; reasons for not using HIVST, etc.].

F: Perceived control towards HIVST
Q9: Think back to your HIV testing experiences or knowledge about HIV testing; What do you think will make it easy for you to do HIVST[**Probe:** training on HIVST; availability of HIVST kits, demonstrations on how to do HIVST, simple /clear instruction, language, etc.].

Q 10: Think back to your HIV testing experiences or knowledge about HIV testing; What do you think will make it hard for you to do HIVST? [**Probe:** risky behaviours (e.g., alcohol/substance abuse; risky sexual behaviours (i.e., unprotected sex; transactional sex; multiple sexual partners)].

G: Barriers to, and facilitators for HIVST
Q11: Think of people who may decide to use **HIVST**; What do you think will motivate or impede them to test for HIV? [**Probe:** lack of policy on **HIVST**; lack of regulatory systems for **HIVST**; lack of knowledge on **HIVST**; lack of counsellor assistance; lack of the **HIVST** kits; fear of HIV-positive results, inability to perform the testing, cost of buying **HIVST** kits, etc.].

H: Self-efficacy towards HIVST
Q12: How confident are you that you would self-test for HIV? [**Probe:** ways to overcome the barriers to HIVST; ways to enhance facilitators for HIVST, etc.].

Q13: In your opinion, how do you think HIVST should be conducted?
[**Probe:** how will this be possible? Someone gets a self-test kit, and then go to test in privacy, then what next? Would they prefer self-testing at the clinic or alternative sites? Provision of assistance from counsellors? A need for post-test counselling? Confirmatory test for HIV positive results? Referral of HIV-positives to care & treatment? , the role of opinion leaders in promoting HIVST intervention, channels of communication, etc.].

CONCLUSION:

Interviewer: Now I have asked you all my questions. Do you have additional comments to increase HIVST uptake or advice on how best to conduct an HIVST intervention at a health facility for at high-risk adults?

Appendix G: Quantitative questionnaire

SECTION A: BACKGROUND INFORMATION OF PARTICIPANTS			
No:	QUESTIONS AND FILTERS	CODING CATEGORIES	SKIP
A.1	Sex	01: Female 02: Male	
A.2	In what date, month and year were you born?	Date of Birth(dd/mm/yyyy):......../......./....../	
A.3	Have you ever attended school?	01: Yes 02: No	**Is the answer is No go to A.5**
A.4	If yes, what is the highest level of school you attended?	01: Primary education 02: Never completed primary education 03: Secondary education 04: Never completed secondary education 05: Higher education	
A.5	What is your religion?	01: Moslem 02: Christian 03: Other denomination	
A.6	What is your marital status?	01: Married (monogamous) 02: Married (polygamous) 03: Co-habiting 04: Single 05: Divorced 06: Widow 07: Widower	
A.7	With whom do you currently live with?	01: Husband/wife 02: A sexual partner 03: A live-in partner 04: Living alone 05: Other (specify)	
A.8	What is your occupation?	01: Female bar worker 02: Porter 03: Other (specify):	
A.9	Which of the following is the main source of your income?	01: My husband/wife/live-in partner 02: Other family members 03: Paid work (seasonal) 04: Paid work (permanent) 05: Own business 06: Sex /commercial work 07: Other (specify):	
SECTION B: RELATIONSHIPS AND SEXUAL HISTORY. This section will assess your relationships and sexual history. We will provide detailed descriptions for sexually related questions. Please answer these questions to your level of understanding.			
Now I would like to ask about your relationships and recent sexual activity. Let me assure you again that your answers are completely confident and will not be revealed to anyone. If we should come to any question that you don't want to answer, just let me know and we will go to the next question.			
B.10	How old where you when you had sexual intercourse for the **first time**?	00: Never had sexual intercourse	**If the answer is**

1

Appendix H: Instructional sheet on how to use HIVST (Swahili version)

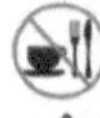

NJIA YA MATUMIZI

Ili upate tokeo sahihi lazima uyafuate maagizo haya kwa makini. Dakika 15 kabla ya upimaji, usile wala kunywa chochote vivyo hivyo usitumie dawa ya meno dakika 30 kabla ya upimaji.

ONYO: Iwapo una Virusi Vya Ukimwi, VVU na unatumia dawa (ART) huenda ukapata tokeo lisilo la kweli, linalo onyesha ati huna virusi.

DIRECTIONS FOR USE

You must follow the test directions carefully to get an accurate result. Do not eat or drink for at least 15 minutes before you start the test or use mouth cleaning products 30 minutes before you start the test.

WARNING: If you are HIV-positive and on HIV treatment (ARVs) you may get a false negative result.

JINSI YA KUTUMIA ORAQUICK, KIPIMA VIRUSI VYA UKIMWI, VVU, CHA KIBINAFSI / HOW TO USE THE OraQuick® HIV SELF-TEST KIT

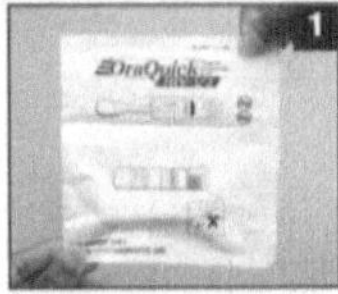

Kipima Virusi chako kina pakiti mbili zilizo unganishwa.
Your test kit contains two pouches.

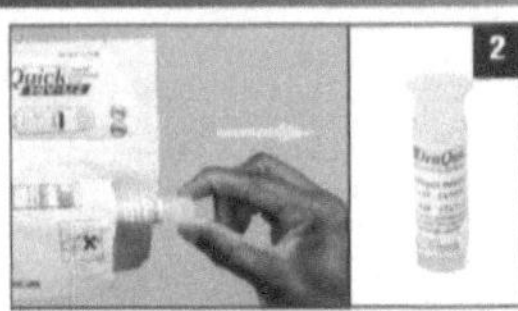

Rarua pakiti upande wenye mchoro wa Kichupa, kisha toa **kichupa.**
Tear open the pouch containing the **tube**.

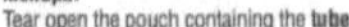

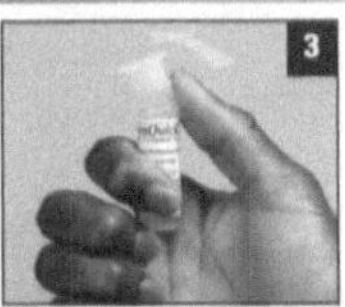

Toa kizibo/kifuniko cha kichupa.
Remove the cap.

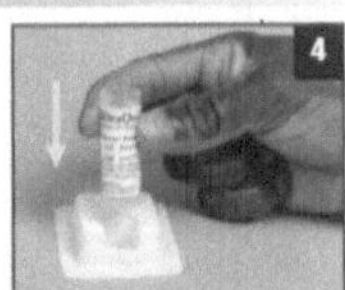

Kalisha kichupa ndani ya **Kikalio**.
Slide the tube into the **stand**.

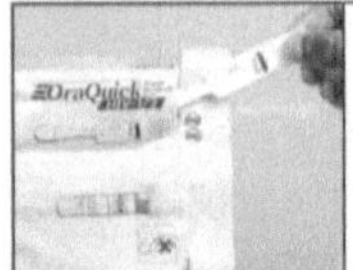

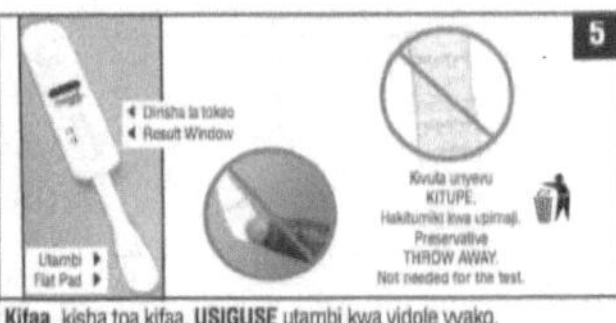

Rarua pakiti upande wenye mchoro wa **Kifaa**, kisha toa kifaa. **USIGUSE** utambi kwa vidole vyako.
Tear open pouch containing the **test device** and remove. **DO NOT** touch the flat pad with your fingers.

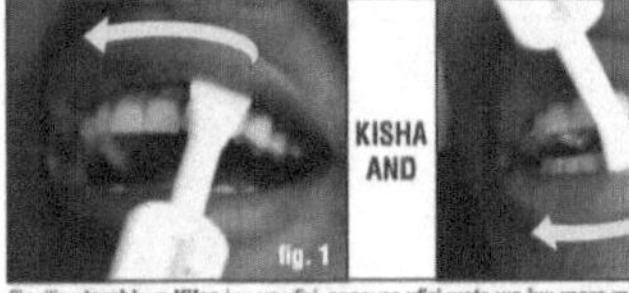

Finyilia **utambi wa Kifaa** juu ya ufizi, pangusa **ufizi wote wa juu mara moja** (fig.1) na pia **ufizi wote wa chini mara moja** (fig.2).
Press the **Flat Pad** firmly against your gum and swab it along your **upper gum once** (fig. 1) and **your lower gum once** (fig. 2).

www.ingramcontent.com/pod-product-compliance
Lightning Source LLC
LaVergne TN
LVHW091153150826
845672LV00005B/1134

* 9 7 8 3 3 8 4 2 7 9 5 4 5 *